The International Library

PROBLEMS IN
PSYCHOPATHOLOGY

Founded by C. K. Ogden

The International Library of Psychology

PSYCHOANALYSIS
In 28 Volumes

PROBLEMS IN
PSYCHOPATHOLOGY

T W MITCHELL

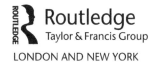

LONDON AND NEW YORK

First published in 1927
by Routledge, Trench, Trubner & Co., Ltd.
2 Park Square, Milton Park, Abingdon, Oxfordshire OX14 4RN
711 Third Avenue, New York, NY 10017

First issued in paperback 2014

Routledge is an imprint of the Taylor and Francis Group, an informa business

British Library Cataloguing in Publication Data
A CIP catalogue record for this book
is available from the British Library

Problems in Psychopathology
ISBN 0415-21102-6
Psychoanalysis: 28 Volumes
ISBN 0415-21132-8
The International Library of Psychology: 204 Volumes
ISBN 0415-19132-7

ISBN 13: 978-1-138-87566-1 (pbk)
ISBN 13: 978-0-415-21102-4 (hbk)

CONTENTS

PRE-FREUDIAN PSYCHOLOGY

PSYCHOLOGY as "science of the soul" has a long history, and speculations on the nature of the soul have seldom been entirely uninfluenced by opinions concerning the nature of the body. We should, therefore, expect to find that men whose vocations or interests led them to have special knowledge of the structure and workings of the body should also have been foremost in speculation about the nature and seat of the soul ; and both the history of medicine and the history of psychology confirm our expectations. Although in modern times specialization has led to a wide divergence of pursuits and interests among those who devote themselves to different branches of knowledge—a divergence almost unknown in the pre-scientific era—the alliance of medicine and psychology, so common in early times, has never quite come to an end, and we may trace the influence of medical science on the theories and practical applications of psychology all through the ages, from Alcmæon of Crotona to Freud of Vienna.

We are, indeed, apt to forget how many of the great psychologists were medical men, or had, at least, studied medicine before they turned towards Psychology and Philosophy. Leaving out of account the medical

1 B

psychologists of ancient times, we may call to mind that John Locke, Hartley, Fechner, Lotze, Wundt, William James, and many others were members of the medical profession ; as, indeed, are also some of the most distinguished psychologists of the present day. Thus it is perhaps not too fanciful to suggest that much that has become incorporated in the body of knowledge sometimes referred to as Academic Psychology, belongs in a sense to Medical Psychology. Putting it in this way at least serves to remind us that the science of Psychology is *one* and that such subdivisions as Medical Psychology, Industrial Psychology, Educational Psychology, are merely abstractions which we make for practical purposes or for convenience in exposition.

Throughout ancient and mediaeval times we find the physiological knowledge of the day controlling, or, at least, greatly influencing, psychological and philosophical speculation. After Galen's time it was commonly accepted that the organs of sense are related to perception, and that the brain is the organ of mind ; and by the end of the sixteenth century mental pathology had advanced so far as to postulate a correlation of cerebral and mental disorder. But the path towards progress in the localization of mental functions in the brain became deflected in the seventeenth century towards a search for the seat of the soul.

In the beginning of the nineteenth century the work of Gall and Spurzheim gave a fresh impetus to investigation of the relations between brain structure and mental processes, and the researches then begun have continued without ceasing up to the present time. The observations of Bouillaud, Broca, and their successors on the cerebral lesions associated with certain defects of speech, and the experimental work on cerebral localization initiated by Fritz and Hitzig and by Ferrier and Horsley, led to a rapid advance in knowledge of the physiology of the brain and spinal cord ; and the data thus obtained had to be taken into consideration by psychologists when dealing with various problems of perception, ideation, volition, and movement. Yet here, as on many former occasions, imperfect observation or unwarranted inference by medical " authorities " led to false notions in psychology. Present-day views of cerebral localization give us a picture very different from that of the sharply defined " centres " of thirty or forty years ago, and the work of Marie, von Monakow, and Henry Head on aphasia has completely revolutionized our conceptions of the relation of cerebral lesion to disorders of speech.

The rapid growth in our knowledge of the anatomy, histology, and physiology of the nervous system in the latter part of the nineteenth century fostered the hope which to-day seems to many of us so vain, that all the phenomena of mental life might ere long be described in terms of cerebral function, and that all mental disorder could be attributed to definite neural lesion. A good deal might here be said about the utilization of physiological data in the formulation of psychological hypotheses, and about the false doctrines in psychology which have been bolstered up by evidence supplied by cerebral pathology; but it is perhaps better to emphasize the scantiness of our knowledge concerning the cerebral correlates of mental processes than to run the risk of suggesting that the little we do know is more important than it actually is. For, above all, it is necessary to guard against the " inveterate habit of confounding the psychical and the physical which is the bane of modern psychology ".[1] In medical psychology as in general psychology we must not be tempted to forget that our immediate object is the investigation of mental states and processes, whatever means we may adopt to attain our ends, or whatever applications we may make of the knowledge so acquired. Even if our knowledge of the structure and the workings of the nervous system were so complete that we could account for every detail of human behaviour in terms of the reflex arc, we should not have learnt anything of psychology proper. Psychology is not a science of neural processes, nor is it the science of behaviour. It is a science of mind. It is the science of the mental accompaniments of the neural processes

[1] James Ward, *Principles of Psychology*, p. 52.

through which behaviour is effected. And in medical psychology it is necessary, perhaps more than in general psychology, to remember that it is a positive science, that it deals with what is, and not with what ought to be, or with what we think ought to be.

From considering the part played by medical science in the history of psychology in so far as physiological and pathological data have been made use of by psychologists, we must turn to another department of medicine—to Medical Psychology itself—if we are to grasp the true nature and the extent of the contribution of Medicine to the science of mind. Medical Psychology is primarily the psychology of abnormal mental states : it is mental pathology or pathological psychology ; when applied to the restoration of disordered mind it is mental therapeutics.

Every science, in its beginnings, passes through a phase of description and classification of the phenomena observed, and up to a quite recent time description and classification were all that had been achieved in mental pathology. Description comes first, and its value depends on the accuracy of observation and clinical acumen of the recorder. Classification is a somewhat later stage, and it must be tentative or provisional until sufficient knowledge has been accumulated. The great clinical observers of the past have left us records in which they described with wonderful accuracy the observable phenomena of

abnormal mental states ; but when they speculated
on the causation or inward meaning of the abnormalities
of thought or behaviour which they described so well
they had little to say which is now of any value. Their
attempts at classification are obsolete, for only within
comparatively recent years has it been possible to
bring any order into the chaos which confronted the
student of abnormal mental states in former times.

The first glimmerings of enlightenment came through
the study of hypnotism. Trance states which occurred
spontaneously had long been known, but only when
trance could be induced artificially, and its course
controlled, did it become possible to add the method of
experiment to that of observation. Investigation was
greatly handicapped by the prejudiced attitude of
men of science, who denied the actuality of the
phenomena reported by the mesmerists and early
hypnotists, or thought they had " explained " them
when they attributed everything to the imagination
of the patient or the credulity of the observer. But
in the course of time some men of independent
judgment who were not deterred by the attitude of
their fellow scientists from recognizing facts when
they were put before them, set themselves to study the
peculiarities of the hypnotic state. At first their
efforts were directed towards finding physiological
explanations of hypnotic phenomena, as when Braid
ascribed the onset of hypnosis to the neuro-muscular

fatigue produced by fixed gazing ; but very soon it became evident that no satisfactory explanation could be given unless mental factors were taken into consideration.

The most important result of all the work done in the investigation of hypnotism was the establishment of the part played by suggestion in the induction of the trance and in the control and direction of hypnotic phenomena. It is true that no explanation of suggestion itself, no understanding of what gives rise to suggesti- bility, was forthcoming ; but the discovery of the power of suggestion provided a key which unlocked the door to much that was formerly mysterious.

In the course of time suggestibility came to be regarded as a normal attribute of the mind, and between the suggestibility of the hypnotic state and the suggestibility of everyday waking life there was thought to be only a difference of degree—a more or less of some quality of mind which still eluded investigation. But it was acknowledged that suggestion in hypnosis had results which could not ordinarily be obtained in the waking state, and, although it was held that the hypnotic state was itself a product of suggestion, nevertheless, it was clear that the establishment of a state of hypnosis did in itself bring about an increase of suggestibility.

Although it might be said that normal suggestibility is all that is requisite for the induction of hypnosis,

yet it was found that certain conditions have usually
to be observed. The subject must be at rest, all
muscular movement being avoided, and the field of
consciousness must be restricted by direction of the
attention to some object or idea and by the inhibition
of all intrusive thoughts   Hypnosis being commonly
regarded as a " sleep " of some kind, suggestions of
sleep are usually employed for the purpose of inducing
the state.

It has long been recognized that such suggestions
may be given in two different ways : either in an
emphatic masterful manner as of one having authority,
or repeated in a soft, coaxing monotone such as a
mother might use when trying to soothe a fretful child.
The relative advantages of the two methods have often
been discussed, and sometimes one, sometimes the other
has been extolled. The origin and significance of these
two ways of giving suggestion were not suspected in
former days, and the success of one rather than the
other, in any particular case, could not be explained.

It was very soon discovered that all suggestions
during hypnosis are not equally effective. Some seem
to be more easily fulfilled than others. For example,
inability to open the eyes, or cataleptic rigidity of
limbs, can be brought about by suggestion in almost
everyone who is at all susceptible to hypnosis, whilst
hallucination and delusions can be induced in only
a relatively small number of people. Various stages or

degrees of hyposis thus came to be recognized, the delimitations of which were determined by the kind of suggestions that are effective in them and by some apparently spontaneous phenomena which appear to be characteristic of each stage or degree. Perhaps the most important dividing line in the series of changes observed as hypnosis becomes deeper is that beyond which the events of hypnosis are forgotten when normal waking life is resumed. Such forgetting— post-hypnotic amnesia as it is called—may arise spontaneously when a certain depth of hypnosis is reached, or it may be brought about by suggestion ; and the degree of hypnosis characterized by post-hypnotic amnesia is technically known as hypnotic somnambulism.

When hypnosis has been induced it is found that some peculiar relation has arisen between the hypnotist and the hypnotized person. It is of such a nature that the subject attends to the words and actions of the hypnotist only ; suggestions given by anyone else are not responded to, and in the deeper stages are not even heard. This is the condition well known to the mesmerists and called by them the state of *rapport*. These early investigators gave a description of *rapport* which contains the essence of what we believe about it to-day ; one of them very aptly compared it to the relation which exists between a sleeping mother and her child : the mother is alert to the slightest sound made by the child, but she is indifferent to all other sounds. In a similar way, the hypnotized person goes to sleep with the thought of the hypnotist in his mind, and during the trance hears only his words. It is obvious, however, that this account will have to be supplemented by some explanation why *rapport* should arise between the subject of experiment and the experimentalist. It will have to be asked, What forces at work in the process of being hypnotized can call forth a relation between two strangers which can be aptly compared to the relation between a sleeping mother and her child ?

In examining the psychological phenomena of hypnotism the first thing to be clearly grasped and never forgetten is that the hypnotic state is always a state of consciousness (awareness). Sometimes, but very rarely, a profoundly lethargic condition occurs in which communication with the subject may present some momentary difficulty ; but for all practical purposes we may regard it as a rule without exception that every genuine hypnosis is a conscious state. In the light stages, before post-hypnotic amnesia occurs or can be produced, there is never any question of the conscious nature of the state. The subject, on awaking, knows that he has been conscious all the time, because he can remember everything that has occurred while he was in the hypnotic state. But when post-hypnotic amnesia is complete, the subject, on being awakened from hypnosis, thinks he must have been unconscious, for he can remember nothing that has happened since the operator told him to sleep. The judgment of onlookers will be different. They have seen him act in response to suggestions, they have heard him reply intelligently to questions, they have observed that his memory of his past life is as good as in his waking state. What they have witnessed compels them to believe that the hypnotized person is conscious all the time, whatever differences from the normal state he may show in other respects.

The belief that a hypnotized person is an unconscious automaton is difficult to account for. Probably its origin may be traced to the preconceptions of the mesmerists, and to the misinterpretation of the evidence which their practice supplied. A hypnotized person is so suggestible, and in many respects so plastic, that if he is treated as an automaton he will behave like one. But, on the other hand, if he is treated as a conscious human being—a method of inquiry strangely neglected by investigators—he will behave like one in almost every respect.

There are, however, some differences almost always noticeable which indicate that the subject is not in his normal waking state. The most striking and most constantly observed difference is the passivity, both bodily and mental, and the lack of spontaneity or initiative shown by the hypnotized person when he is not asked to speak or to act. In the course of conversation with him he must be stimulated by questions or remarks ; if the operator ceases to ask questions or to make comments, the subject soon relapses into silence. It may be laid down as a general rule that a hypnotized person does not speak and does not act, unless he is directly or indirectly asked to do so.

When a person is hypnotized for the first time and a degree of hypnosis is obtained which makes it possible to inhibit certain voluntary movements, although no other experimental suggestions are effective, we find that we are dealing with a person whose mental state is extremely interesting. So long as no inhibitory suggestions are given to him, it is difficult to find evidence that his mental condition is in any way abnormal. He is perhaps unusually still and shows no inclination to make any spontaneous movements ; but if he is questioned—and with care this may be done without disturbing the hypnosis—he will appear to be his normal self. But corresponding to the bodily restfulness there appears to be some immobility of the mind. During the hypnotizing process his attention was fixed on the operator and while the state lasts this direction of attention persists. He is consequently disinclined to pay any regard to stimuli from other sources which normally would attract his attention. The conversation of other people who may be present is heard, but unless their remarks are about himself he tends to disregard them. This attitude is exhibited more clearly in the deeper stages which border on somnambulism.

So long, then, as no inhibitory suggestions are given, there is little to be discovered in the mental state of a person in the lighter degrees of hypnosis which would lead us to suppose that it differed from what is to be found in normal waking life. But when such a suggestion is given and is effective, it is immediately clear that something unusual has happened. I extend the arm of a hypnotized person and say : " You cannot bend your arm." If now I ask him to try to bend his arm, various results may be observed. Perhaps the most common and most interesting result is that he makes a seemingly determined effort to bend the arm. The hand is acutely flexed at the wrist, a look of mingled perplexity and amusement comes over his face, and he finally confesses that he cannot bend the arm. Sometimes, however, apparently no attempt to do so is made ; he simply confesses at once that he cannot do it. At other times the effort is successful although evidently with difficulty ; the flexor muscles are powerfully contracted and after a short struggle the opposing muscles give way.

The state of mind underlying suggested immobility of this kind is of extraordinary interest, and is of paramount importance for the understanding of the nature of hypnotic suggestibility. The most commonly accepted interpretation of such phenomena is that they are examples of ideo-motor action. It is supposed that the mental state of a hypnotized person is such that every idea suggested by the operator infallibly works itself out in appropriate action, uninfluenced by the will or personality of the subject. It is vaguely recognized that the fulfilment of a suggestion implies that the suggested idea has been in some sense " accepted " ; and it is said that when a suggestion is not fulfilled, it is not fulfilled because it is not accepted, and that it is not accepted because hypnosis is not sufficiently deep for that particular suggestion. But if we use the word accept in its ordinary sense we may say that not every suggestion that is accepted can be fulfilled, although every suggestion that is fulfilled must have been accepted. To accept an idea is not merely to have an idea and to understand it, it is to assent to it ; and assent to a proposition presented to a hypnotized person is not compelled by the mere assertion of the hypnotist. This has been demonstrated on many occasions in regard to suggestions that are opposed to the hypnotized person's ideas of what is right and proper ; and whilst there is much evidence that suggestions of this kind are rejected, just as they would be in waking life, there is no proof that suggestions are ever accepted in hypnosis that would not be accepted, at least as " make believe ", in the ordinary waking state.

We must conclude, then, that the suggestion " You cannot bend your arm ", has been accepted in the sense of being assented to ; and the state of the subject's mind, when he apparently does try hard to perform the inhibited movement, probably finds its best parallel in the normal state during the performance of such an experiment as that which William James described as follows : " Try to feel as if you were crooking your finger, whilst keeping it straight. In a minute it will fairly tingle with the imaginary change of position ; yet it will not sensibly move, because *its not really moving* is also a part of what you have in mind. Drop *this* idea, think of the movement purely and simply, with all breaks off ; and presto ! it takes place with no effort at all." [1]

Now, to drop the inhibitory idea is just what the hypnotized person seems unable to do. He has assented to the suggestion that he cannot bend his arm, and he cannot, or he will not, let it go when the idea of bending his arm arises. Assent to the inhibitory suggestion may be, and generally is, a mere acquiescence in the request or command of the hypnotist ; but the fulfil-ment of the suggestion, the rigidity of the arm, bears the marks of a willed movement, or, at least, of some form of conation. Yet on the surface it would seem as if the whole voluntary effort of the hypnotized person were directed towards the overcoming of the suggested

[1] *Principles of Psychology*, vol. ii, p. 527.

fixation of his arm, and since the effort is unavailing it is natural to suppose that his arm has been rendered rigid against his will. But if we look a little deeper we may see that the fixation of the arm is the action that is really willed, and we may recognize that we have in such experiments the beginnings of that division of the self which reaches such extraordinary development in the various forms of double personality.

Suggested rigidity in the hypnotic state resembles the voluntary action of a self that cannot bend the arm because it will not. If by suggestion the rigidity be prolonged into the waking state, we have then a self that does not bend the arm because it cannot. Only when the hypnotic self is willing does the waking self regain control of the inhibited movement.

A profoundly significant reply is frequently given by hypnotized persons when they are challenged to perform some movement that has been inhibited by suggestion. They say : " I feel I don't want to." This seems to be the true psychological explanation of the efficacy of inhibitory suggestion in hypnosis, and of many of the so-called uncontrollable aberrations of conduct in ordinary life. In both cases those who realize at once that they don't want to, do not try ; and those who appear to try but do not succeed don't really want to either.

Hypnotic states, besides showing increased suggestibility, reveal some peculiarities of the memory function, which are interesting and instructive. Some of these are an immediate result of the onset of hypnosis, some are the product of direct or indirect suggestion during hypnosis, and some are related to the emergence from hypnosis and the return to the normal waking state.

On passing into hypnosis the range of recollection is increased so that memories can be recalled which do not come into consciousness in the waking state. Recollections of this kind may be facilitated by suggestion during hypnosis, and the deeper the hypnosis the more extensive does the memory become. This is especially true of events in the past life of the hypnotized person. Incidents of childhood which have been long lost to memory may come to the surface, or more recent events which were accompanied by much emotional disturbance and subsequently forgotten may be recovered.

In the deep stage, known as hypnotic somnambulism, this power of recollection is at its highest, yet when the hypnotized person is awakened from the trance state all memory of the events that have happened during hypnosis seems to have vanished; not only have the recovered memories disappeared, apparently beyond recall, but there is also complete oblivion of all that has been said or done during the somnambulism. But, although such loss of recollection might appear to be the natural and inevitable consequence of somnambulism, it is noteworthy that it can be entirely avoided by the simple expedient of giving to the hypnotized person a suggestion that all the events of the trance state shall be remembered on awaking. This possibility of annulling post-hypnotic amnesia by suggestion raises important problems concerning the nature of the forces at work in the production of such forgetfulness and such suggestibility.

What was learnt about suggestion and amnesia from the study of hypnotism was corroborated by the investigation of hysteria. In this malady the peculiarities of mental and bodily function which can be produced by suggestion during hypnosis are found to occur spontaneously, and, since they may persist as symptoms of the disorder for relatively long periods, they are in some ways better suited for investigation than are the more ephemeral phenomena of hypnotism.

The suggestibility of the hysteric has become a by-word, and some writers have gone so far as to say that all people who are suggestible are in so far forth hysterical. Suggestibility is regarded as one of the stigmata of hysteria, and since the symptoms of hysteria can be produced by suggestion, it has also been said that all hysteria is nothing but suggestion. For the present we need not stop to examine these assertions or to inquire into the differences, if any there be, between hypnosis and hysteria ; all that is necessary is to look at some of the similarities and to get what light we can on their mechanism and significance.

In hysteria somnambulisms sometimes occur which seem to stand in the same relation to the normal consciousness as does hypnotic somnambulism ; that is to say, there is no recollection of the events of the trance state when normal life is resumed. These somnambulisms may occur in the form of hysterical attacks of short duration, or they may take the form of fugues, lasting for days or weeks, in which the patient forgets who he is, wanders from home and friends, lives with strangers, and takes up new interests which seem alien to his known character. More rarely there is a true doubling of personality in which two or more phases of consciousness, each having the characteristics of personality, alternate one with another. The memory relations of the alternating phases are not the same in all forms of double personality. Sometimes there is reciprocal amnesia, so that in each phase there is no recollection of the other. Sometimes the amnesia affects one phase only, the other having clear recollection of the experiences of the phase with which it alternates. The form in which the memory relations most closely resemble those of hypnotic somnambulism is that known as the co-conscious type of double personality. In this form the secondary personality has recollection of the experiences of the primary, and presumably normal, personality, but the primary personality has no recollection of the experiences of the secondary one.

All forms of somnambulism have been ascribed to a splitting of the mind whereby a smaller system of ideas becomes dissociated from the larger system constituting personality. This is the essence of the explanation put forward by Professor Janet many years ago, adhered to by him up to the present time, and accepted in a general way by the great majority of psychologists. According to this view, both the suggestibility and the amnesia of hysteria and hypnosis are direct and inevitable consequences of dissociation. Just because the suggested idea or the dissociated system remains isolated from the system of ideas which form the personal consciousness, it is free from the restraining influence which these ideas would exert, and is able to develop to its full extent ; hence the almost supernormal force which suggestion seems to have and the compulsive nature of somnambulic acts. So, also, just because the experiences of somnambulism are dissociated from the personal consciousness, there is complete forgetfulness of these experiences when the trance comes to an end.

An interesting feature of Janet's conception of somnambulism is the parallel he draws between the somnambulic fit and all other hysterical manifestations. Far from considering somnambulism as a rare phenomenon, he looks upon it as the most characteristic symptom of hysteria and the type on which all other hysterical symptoms are modelled. Anæsthesia and paralysis, disturbances of the special senses, disorders of the great functional systems of the body, and, indeed, all hysterical manifestations whatsoever, are of the nature of somnambulism inasmuch as they are the outcome of dissociations of systems of sensations and images which continue to function outside the personal consciousness. Janet describes the occurrence of dissociation to lack of a hypothetical psychical tension which normally keeps the mind a synthetic unity. According to his most recent writings, it would seem that he considers almost all the phenomena of disordered mental life to be dependent upon, or related to, the rise and fall of psychical tension. But he also introduces another factor which must be taken into account if we are to understand why lack of psychical tension bears upon certain elements of mental life rather than upon others. The mind includes a great variety of tendencies and capacities, some of which are well organized and stable, whilst others, of more recent acquisition, are less firmly organized and more liable to disturbance. There is a hierarchy of mental functions, at each ascending level of which a higher and higher degree of tension is necessary. The more difficult and complex an act is, the greater is the tension required for its proper performance ; the easier and simpler it is the less tension is necessary. When the

tide of psychical tension falls too low and the stress of
life is too great, the most recent acquisitions, the most
difficult and complex activities, are the first to suffer.

Janet is here applying to mental functions the conceptions put forward by Hughlings Jackson in his
lectures " On the Evolution and Dissolution of the
Nervous System ". The value and importance of this
general conception is undoubted ; it is the law of
dissolution wherever in nature this process occurs.
But disintegration is not always by way of dissolution ;
it may be due to stress from without or stress
from within which falls unevenly on the integrated
system, and when this happens loss of function may
not follow in regression the path laid down in evolution.
Indeed, Janet himself has found that a general lowering
of psychical tension does not lead to the production
of the phenomena most characteristic of hysteria,
but to those of another great group of mental disorders which he classifies under the general term
Psychasthenia. Among the symptoms of psychasthenia
he includes obsessions, doubts, compulsions, phobias,
anxiety states, feelings of incompleteness, and
depersonalization. In psychasthenia he sees the results
of a general lowering of all the mental functions,
especially of the highest, but in hysteria there is a
localization of the mental insufficiency on one or other
particular function. The lowering of the level of
psychical tension leads here to a retraction of the field

of consciousness, not, except in a minor degree, to a general diminution of function. When the mental operations or the acts to be performed are too complex and too difficult, consciousness loses grip of them altogether, and they become dissociated.

Always, in his elucidation of the nature and mechanism of hysteria, Janet is faced with this problem of localization. " How is it," he asks, " that with one person the hysteria bears on the arm, with another on the stomach, and that with a third it only reaches a system of ideas, which it turns into a somnambulism." To this question he gives no satisfactory answer. Sometimes he says localization may be determined by suggestion or by some process akin to suggestion, but not identical with it ; sometimes by the function on which dissociation bears having remained weak and disturbed " for some reason or other " ; sometimes by the function that disappears having been the most complicated and the most difficult for the subject ; sometimes by the function having been in full activity at the moment of a great emotion. Behind these answers there lie some deeper problems which he leaves unsolved, for example, why did the function affected remain weak and disturbed ? Why was it the most complicated and difficult *for the subject ?*

In Janet's theory of hysteria and psychasthenia we have a purely mechanical conception of the forces at work in the integration and disintegration of the personal life. It does not take into consideration any forces within the self other than the vague force referred to as psychical tension. It leaves the symptoms devoid of all meaning and unrelated to the conative and affective experience of the patient in the past or in the present. If we start with a mechanically determined dissociation as the primary factor in the production of abnormalities of thought and conduct, we must end without vision of the meaning and significance of these abnormalities, if meaning and significance they have.

FREUD AND PSYCHO-ANALYSIS

TOWARDS the close of the nineteenth century a solitary scientific worker, Sigmund Freud, of Vienna, discovered a new method of investigating the human mind—the method of Psycho-analysis. As a result of his work on hysteria and allied disorders, he arrived at conclusions so novel and so surprising, so unwelcome and so wounding to man's self-esteem, that for many years his views were almost entirely ignored or rejected with scorn and indignation. The pioneers of hypnotism had met with somewhat similar treatment, and yet, as we have seen, their work was the first to shed any light on the problems of medical psychology. And now we can see that the work of Freud, and the new method in psychology which he originated, have led to an illumination of mental process, both abnormal and normal, which but a few years ago could not have been thought possible of attainment in our time.

It does not need much courage to express such a conviction to-day, for it is a conviction held by many of the ablest and most earnest workers in the field of psychopathology and by some eminent psychologists whose work does not lie in the special sphere of the abnormal. But to propound his views and to maintain them single-handed for so many years in the face of

world-wide disbelief and disapprobation did require
courage of a most unusual kind in the founder of
Psycho-analysis. Why psycho-analysis should have
met with so much opposition can be fully explained
only in the light of knowledge derived from psycho-
analysis itself. Indeed, we know that the kind of
reception it had is evidence in support of the truth of
its doctrines. Had it been received with acclamation,
what it taught about the mind could not be true. Had
its doctrines been false, they *might* have been rejected ;
if they were true, rejection was inevitable.

In his early investigations of hysteria Freud worked
in collaboration with another Viennese physician,
Josef Breuer, who, while Freud was still a medical
student, had made the notable discovery that
symptoms of hysteria are in some way related to certain
events in the past life of the patient, that these events
have been forgotten, and that if they can be restored
to memory the symptoms disappear. For the purpose
of recovering these lost memories Breuer took
advantage of the increased power of recollection
manifested in the hypnotic state, and he found that
when the lost memories came back into consciousness
during hypnosis they did so with much vividness
and were accompanied by a great display of feeling.
The beneficial result which accrued to the patient was
ascribed to the outlet thus afforded for pent-up feelings
which had not found expression at the time of

the traumatic episode; and this way of treating hysteria was called by Breuer the *cathartic method*.

Breuer believed that the absence of these memories from the waking consciousness, and the possibility of their recall in hypnosis, were due to the pathogenic experiences having occurred during states of dissociation in some ways resembling hypnosis—conditions of abstraction, or day-dreaming, which he termed *hypnoid states*. A disposition to the occurrence of such states he considered to be an essential feature of the hysterical constitution.

Freud's investigation led him to depart from this somewhat mechanical conception of the genesis of hysteria ; for it seemed to him that in every case he examined he could discern forces at work in the patient's mind which might account for the dissociation and amnesia without any need to postulate the occurrence of hypnoid states. Dissociation appeared to Freud to be due to a forcible rejection of painful thoughts—a process which he described as a defence reaction of the mind against ideas that are unbearable. It was not, however, until he gave up using hypnosis as a means of recovering lost memories that this conception of the origin of dissociation and amnesia came to full fruition.

Breuer's method of investigating and treating hysterical symptoms necessitated having the patient in a state of deep hypnosis. But many neurotic

sufferers cannot be hypnotized, and Freud resolved
to make the method independent of hypnotism. He
had seen Bernheim bring back to memory the events
of deep hypnosis by simply assuring the patient in
the waking state that he could and would remember,
and he resolved to use Bernheim's method as a means
of recovering the lost memories of neurotic patients
who had not been hypnotized. When the patient's
efforts to remember failed, Freud would assure him
that the correct memory would come back at the
moment he pressed his hand on the patient's forehead.
This plan was afterwards referred to as the *pressure
method*.

The reasoning which led Freud to think that what
applies to persons who have been hypnotized must
also apply to those who have not been hypnotized
may seem at first sight not very sound ; for if the
assurances given by Bernheim to his patients, that they
could and would remember the events of a recent
somnambulism, had been given by some other person,
such assurances would not have enabled the patient
to recall the forgotten events. It is the peculiar relation
existing between the person who has been hypnotized
and the person who has hypnotized him which alone
makes possible the efficacy of such assertions as " now
you can remember ". The fact, however, that Freud
by employing this method did succeed in " learning
from the patient all that was necessary for a con-

struction of the connexion between the forgotten pathogenic scenes and the symptoms which they had left behind " is sufficient proof that in the process of analysis some relation arises between patient and analyst which is similar to the *rapport* of hypnosis.

Although this method succeeded in Freud's hands, it must not be supposed that the forgotten memories were easily recovered. The correct thoughts did not always come when pressure was made and great perseverance was necessary in carrying out analysis in this way. Freud tells us that he found the method very exhausting and that it seemed to him as if the memories were being kept back by some force, some resistance, against which he had to struggle if the patient was to be cured. At this point Freud had one of those flashes of inspiration which are the hall mark of genius. This force, he thought, which now appears as resistance to recall, must be the very force which originally caused the forgetting ; what keeps these memories out of consciousness now must have been the cause of their exclusion from consciousness from the beginning. Thus arose Freud's great conception of *repression* [1] as being the immediate cause of dissociation and amnesia—a conception which forms the foundation stone on which the whole structure of psycho-analysis rests.

[1] A technical term, defined later, which must not be confused with repression in its ordinary connotation, e.g. checking.

A general indication of the nature of the forces at work in repression was obtained from an examination of the kind of experiences which were forgotten by the patients he had treated. In every case he found that the things that could not voluntarily be recalled were things which caused unpleasant feelings when they were by any means brought back into consciousness. They were always related to some wish which had arisen in the patient's mind and had come into conflict with his ethical or æsthetic ideals. The mechanism of hysterical symptoms began to be clear. It seemed to derive its motive power from a series of mental events—first of all an unacceptable wish, then mental conflict, then repression, and, finally, symptom formation. Each member of this series gave rise to fresh problems, some of which are not yet fully solved : (1) What kind of wishes or ideas are so unacceptable to neurotic patients that they are rejected and repressed ? (2) What can we learn about the nature and origin of the forces opposed to the repressed wishes ? (3) What happens to the rejected ideas or wishes when they are repressed ? (4) What is the connexion between the repressed wishes and the symptoms ?

(1) The pressure method of recovering lost memories was not adhered to for long, and Breuer's plan of starting with the investigation of particular symptoms was also give up. Every case examined showed how complex is the structure of a neurosis, and it became

plain that nothing short of analysis of the whole mind would reveal all the determinants of the symptoms.

The patient was allowed to tell his story in his own way provided that he undertook to say everything that came into his mind without reservation and without selection or rejection of the incoming thoughts. This was a hard task for the patient, because some things came into his mind which he did not care to tell, and he often had to be reminded of his promise to tell all ; but as the analysis went on his natural unwillingness to reveal his most intimate thoughts was overcome, and, if he was in earnest about his recovery, he soon was able to tell any thoughts of which he himself was clearly conscious. But this was only a preliminary and superficial difficulty : the real difficulty was to bring back into clear consciousness the thoughts and feelings that had been repressed. The forces which had caused the repression were still at work, and in spite of the good will of the patient they still prevented the return of the lost memories. Much that came into his mind did not appear to have any connexion with his illness, and memories arose which, on the surface, at least, seemed quite irrelevant. But Freud believed that every mental process is determined, and he could not avoid the conviction that the seemingly irrelevant thoughts were related, in some way, to the repressed thoughts which he was seeking. And he found that this was so. The seemingly irrelevant thoughts, when they were used as the starting point for further free association proved to be of the nature of allusions, more or less direct, to the revelant thoughts which ultimately emerged. The resistance which in the pressure method he had felt as a force against which he had to struggle now came to light in the devious course taken by the associations before the repressed thoughts could be recovered. Indeed, the indirectness of the allusions could be taken as a measure of the resistance.

When a patient is allowed to tell his story in his own way, it is found that there are many gaps in the narrative which he relates. Some of these are omissions of experiences which for the moment he has forgotten, although they are experiences which he is quite able to recall. Some of the gaps, however, are due to omission of experiences, memories of which *do* come into consciousness during the narrative, but are kept back because the telling of them would be painful or embarrassing to the patient. It becomes plain, however, that there are some gaps in the narrative which the patient is unable to fill up by any voluntary effort.

It is noteworthy that the thoughts deliberately kept back or suppressed are those which the patient is ashamed to tell, for investigation of the causes of both the temporary and the persistent lapses of memory revealed in the narrative leads to the conclusion that here also feelings like shame and disgust are concerned in keeping away from consciousness the things that are forgotten.

The resistance revealed in a patient's first account of his illness becomes more clearly obvious when analysis is undertaken. The associations play around some forgotten experience, recollection of which, when the memory does come back, is accompanied by some painful affect. Most frequently, from the very beginning of the analysis, these memories are related to the most intimate experiences of the personal life, above all to the love-life and to those aspects of the love-life which are specifically called sexual. At first the memories recalled may be of recent experiences, but they are found to have associative connexions with earlier experiences of a similar nature dating back perhaps to the time of puberty. But puberty, although it is a period of great bodily and mental transformation, it is not a time of new beginnings ; there is no sharp discontinuity between pre- and post-pubertal life. The experiences of adolescence have manifold associations with experiences of childhood, and these latter are accompanied by feelings having the same quality of pleasure or pain as have the feelings aroused by the related experiences of later life. And so it is found that the specifically sexual experiences of adults have associative connexions with infantile experiences which it has not been customary to call sexual. Yet these infantile experiences are the outcome of

D

tendencies in the child's nature which lead to conduct that is under the same ban of social disapproval as that by which we seek to guard the sexual morality of grown-up people.

These infantile tendencies reveal themselves in conduct which takes the form of finding pleasure in sensations derived from various sensitive parts of the body, in the performance or the witnessing of excretory acts, in curiosity about, and display of, the bodily organs concerned in such acts, and sometimes in the exercise of mastery or the infliction of pain.   The connexion constantly found in analysis between these activities of childhood and the sexual experiences of adult life, combined with the noteworthy fact that when such infantile activities are continued after puberty or reverted to in later life they are un-hesitatingly regarded as sexual perversions, led Freud to the conviction that all such activities, at all ages, carry with them something of a definitely sexual nature.

(2) Such being the source of the experiences from which the content of the forgotten memories of neurotic patients is derived, it might be supposed that the next question to be solved would have been that con-cerning the nature and origin of the forces with which this forgotten material had come into conflict, and by which, presumably, it had been repressed.   This question, however, remained for many years unsolved,

and almost uninvestigated ;   for various reasons a
working hypothesis formulated in very general terms
was all that could be achieved.   It was apparent that
the repressed wishes had met with some stronger forces
in the mind, and these latter were supposed to emanate
from the *Ego*, whereas the forces that were overcome
were derived from the sexual instinct.   Thus a
distinction was set up from the beginning between
Ego-tendencies and sexual tendencies ; but for a long
time analysts were almost entirely occupied with the
investigation of the latter, and only within the last
few years have they begun to undertake a detailed
analysis of the Ego.

It is perhaps unfortunate that these uninvestigated
forces should have been so readily accredited to the
Ego and identified with it, without any very clear
indication being given of what we are to understand
by the Ego or what relation is supposed to obtain
between the Ego of psycho-analysis and the Ego of
former psychologies and philosophies. Being frequently
pressed by their opponents to define these Ego-forces
more precisely and to indicate their source, the psycho-
analysts, again perhaps rather hastily, fell back on the
biological division of instincts into those of self-
preservation and reproduction, and made this biological
division the basis of their psychological distinction
between Ego-instincts and sexual instincts.   But it
was not always clear that the repressing forces are

derived from the instincts usually included in the self-
preservation group, nor was it commonly admitted that
the sexual instincts are so completely divorced from the
Ego as the psycho-analytical antithesis would imply.
It seemed obvious that there was need for a thorough
examination of the concepts denoted by such terms as
Ego, sexual, instinct, etc. But for practical purposes
the meaning of the term Ego as used by psycho-analysts
was plain enough. The Ego comprises all the forces in
the mind that are opposed to the sexual instincts.
These forces include all that is derived from the moral
tradition of civilization, from the effects of cultural
training and education, and from the development of
the æsthetic sense. They are brought into play by
emotions aroused by social disapproval, by that product of social disapproval which is felt as conscience,
and by æsthetic disapproval manifested as loathing
or disgust.

(3) We thus reach the point of understanding in a
general way how the losses of memory met with in
neurotic patients are brought about. Sexual wishes
of some kind, and the ideas associated with them,
come into conflict with wishes of the Ego, and the
result of the conflict is that the wishes and ideas
unacceptable to the Ego are repressed. In what, then
does this act of repression consist ? What happens to
the rejected ideas ? Obviously they are not annihilated
or destroyed, for if they were they would cause no

further trouble ; and all our certain knowledge of the neuroses teaches us that these repressed ideas are directly concerned in their causation. Moreover, we know that the lost memories can be recovered. Where, then, have they been in the meantime ? Have they been " out of mind " in the literal sense of the words ? Have they existed merely as neural dispositions, physical imprints on the brain which need the flashlight of consciousness to bring them back into the mind ? Or have they been in the mind all the time and only lacked the quality of consciousness ?

This is part of an old problem. These questions may be asked about any experience, whether repressed or not, which is not in consciousness at the moment. In every instance of mental retention and recall we may ask, What is the nature of the persisting conditions which we must assume in order to account for the fact of recollection ? The most commonly accepted hypothesis is that every mental event leaves some trace which becomes active again whenever the proper stimulus is given. These traces may be thought of as being either mental or physical, and since the facts of recollection can be equally well explained on either hypothesis it is perhaps of no practical importance whether we conceive traces to be persistent modifications of mind or ultra-microscopic alterations in the substance of the brain. But, if we must assume persistent traces of some kind, it is better, if only on

methodological grounds, to ascribe them to the mind
rather than to the brain ; and the reasons for doing so
are more cogent when we are dealing with the data
of psycho-analysis than when we are merely trying to
account for the phenomena of normal retention and
recall.   For the hypothesis of brain - traces would
seem to suggest that when these traces are not
implicated in any conscious mental event or process
they are entirely passive, and that only when they are
reanimated by perceptual or associational stimuli, and
again form part of the physical substratum of conscious
thought, do they take any part in the work of the mind.
But although such a static rôle may suffice for
the mnemonic phenomena of registration, retention,
and recollection, it seems quite inadequate when we
consider those mental events that seem to be products
of mental activity which has not been conscious. The
static view of brain-traces has then to be supplemented
by some sort of " unconscious cerebration " which does
mental work in the absence of mind. If we accept a
theory of brain-traces and at the same time hold that
only that which is conscious is mental, the data of
psycho-analysis will compel us to believe in the continuous action of " unconscious cerebration ".   And
even if we adopt a theory of mental traces, but still
adhere to the view that only the conscious is mental,
we are compelled to ascribe activity and *some* degree
of consciousness to the traces that enter into the mental

processes which, on the former hypothesis, are ascribed to " unconscious cerebration ". Something of this kind is implied in the doctrine of *subconsciousness* put forward by the late Professor James Ward. It would seem much simpler, and more in accordance with all the facts, to accept the hypothesis of mental dispositions and traces and at the same time to recognize that these are not mere passive imprints on the mind, but that they enter into active relations with each other and supply the content of truly unconscious thought.

The difficulty of understanding how the mind can retain traces and dispositions which become active in unconscious mental process can be got over if we rid ourselves of the old notion that consciousness—the " waking " consciousness of every-day life—is the essence of everything mental. And this should not be difficult ; for there is much evidence that mental events and processes occur which are not open to introspection and never enter consciousness at all. Some of this evidence may be found in examining the normal workings of the mind. The phenomena of post-hypnotic suggestion give incontrovertible proof of the occurrence of non-introspectible mental events. The data of psycho-analysis can hardly be stated or understood unless we assume the occurrence of unconscious mental processes.

An experience that has passed out of consciousness may be regarded as still existing in the mind in the form of a mental trace, and, since the experience is not in consciousness at the moment and yet is in the mind, it may be said to be in unconsciousness. But we have seen that while some things that are unconscious at any moment can easily be brought back into consciousness, other things, for example, the lost memories of hysteria, cannot be recalled by any ordinary means. A distinction must be made between these two ways of being unconscious, and Freud has proposed the term *Preconscious* for all that can be easily recalled, and the term *Unconscious* for all that cannot be recalled, or that can be recalled only by the use of special measures, such as hypnosis or psycho-analysis.

A similar distinction has recently been made by Dr. C. D. Broad, who calls preconscious memories *accessible*, and unconscious memories *inaccessible*. He says : " An experience is accessible when it can be remembered by normal means. It is inaccessible when it can be remembered only, if at all, by special technical methods." [1] The lost memories of hysteria, the experiences which are remembered only after the resistances have been removed by the induction of hypnosis or in the course of analysis, belong to the class which Dr. Broad calls inaccessible ; and he admits that " the work of the psycho-analysts enables us to state one at least of the causes which tend to make

[1] *The Mind and its Place in Nature*, p. 362.

certain experiences inaccessible ". He is here referring
to the Freudian theory of repression. It is sometimes
supposed that a memory tends to become inaccessible
because of the painfulness of the affect which
accompanied the original experience, but as Dr. Broad
very truly says : " The essential factor is the emotional
effect which the *memory* of the experience *would*
have if it arose *now*."   This is exactly what Freud
has taught us, and it is the explanation of the
resistance met with in analysis when we try to recover
the lost memories of hysteria or other neuroses. As
has been already pointed out, the truly pathogenic
memories are to be found in every case far back in
childhood, and they are often memories of experiences
which were by no means unpleasant to the child ;
and when Dr. Broad says that " the memory of many
experiences which were quite enjoyable when they
happened might be shocking or painful to the present
self ", he is giving the explanation, perhaps unwittingly,
why infantile sexuality plays so important a part in
the causation of the neuroses, and why the pleasurable
experiences of childhood are so inaccessible in
adult life.

   We say then that when repression occurs certain
experiences which may have been originally pleasant
have now become unpleasant or painful ; they are
pushed out of consciousness, and they are kept out
of consciousness because of the pain which remem-

brance of them would entail. But repression means more than this. Some things which we may have no right to call experiences at all, for they have never been consciously experienced, are from the beginning kept out of consciousness by repression, just because their entry into consciousness would be accompanied by pain or unpleasure.

There seems to be widespread misapprehension of the nature of repression and of its relation to the unconscious or inaccessible parts of the mind. Even Mr. Bertrand Russell, in his *Analysis of Mind*, falls into the common error of supposing that Freud teaches " that every unconscious wish was once conscious, and was then, in his terminology, ' repressed ' because we disapproved of it. On the contrary," Mr. Russell continues, " we shall suppose that, although Freudian ' repression ' undoubtedly occurs and is important, it is not the usual reason for unconsciousness of our wishes. The usual reason is merely that wishes are all, to begin with, unconscious, and only become known when they are actively noticed." [1]   Now, what Mr. Russell here supposes to be Freud's view is exactly the opposite of what Freud teaches. He has never said or implied that every unconscious wish was once conscious; on the contrary, he believes, with Mr. Russell, " that wishes are all, to begin with, unconscious, and only become known when they are

[1] *The Analysis of Mind*, p. 38.

actively noticed." Where he possibly differs from Mr. Russell is in believing that wishes would not remain unnoticed were it not for the action of the repressing forces which prevents their admission into consciousness. Freud considers all mental processes to be in themselves unconscious and he believes that a mental act commonly goes through two phases, between which is interposed a kind of testing process whereby it is subjected to a scrutiny by that part of the Ego which is the source of the repressing forces. If it is rejected it is repressed and does not pass into the second phase ; if it is not rejected it does pass into the second phase ; it becomes preconscious and thus capable of entering consciousness. It may now, in Mr. Russell's words, " become known " when it is " actively noticed ". According to Freud, " everything that is repressed must remain unconscious, but . . . the repressed does not comprise the whole unconscious. The unconscious has the greater compass : the repressed is a part of the unconscious."

(4) Although everything that is repressed must remain unconscious, it sometimes happens that repression is not entirely successful. The experiences which the neurotic patient finds so hard to remember are linked up with strong unconscious desires or wishes which are always striving to get into consciousness and to achieve satisfaction. The driving force behind them

---

[1] *Collected Papers*, vol. iv, p. 98.

is so powerful that the repressing forces are sometimes unable to keep these wishes wholly in check, and in the end they are admitted into consciousness and allowed gratification, provided that they are distorted or disguised in such a way that neither the nature of the wish nor the nature of the gratification is recognized for what it really is. Analysis has shown very clearly that hysterical symptoms arise in this way, and that they are disguised gratifications of repressed wishes. They are more than this, however ; the Ego-wishes also enter into their formation, and the symptoms represent a compromise between the opposed tendencies.

The fundamental conception of the psycho-analytic theory of neurotic symptom-formation—a conception which was implicit in Janet's early work, but which in its explicit form we really owe to Breuer—is, that neurotic symptoms have meaning. Their meaning, like the meaning of dreams, can only be discerned when they are interpreted. Indeed, the mental processes through which they come into being are the same as, or closely resemble, those that lead to the formation of dreams.

In analysing a dream by the method of free association it is found that a single element in the dream may lead to a great number of unconscious thoughts. In the process of dream-making these thoughts have suffered *condensation*, so that they are all repre-

sented in the single dream-element analysed. Another
mechanism of dream-making is known as *displacement*.
Here some unconscious thought may be represented
in the dream by an indirect allusion which would not
have suggested itself to the waking consciousness as
a suitable substitute ; or the most important element
in the unconscious thought may be but feebly represented in the dream, while an unimportant element
may be strongly emphasized. Another source of the
disguise of unconscious thoughts in dreams is their
appearance in symbolic form—a form not imposed upon
them by the censorship of the Ego, but a form which
unconscious thinking habitually takes.

These are some of the ways in which unconscious
wishes are disguised so that when they are gratified
in dream their significance is not realized by the
dreamer ; and all these mechanisms come into play
in the formation of symptoms. The symptom is
a disguised or symbolic representation of repressed
impulses or wishes. By condensation and displacement it becomes possible for the symptom to stand for
both the unconscious wish and the opposing wish
emanating from the Ego, and thus to serve the purpose
of a compromise.

The meaning of a symptom is always unconscious
and only because its meaning is unconscious is it
possible for a symptom to arise. If the mental process
which gives meaning to a symptom were a conscious

process, no symptom could appear ; and if we can make
the meaning of a symptom conscious, or rather, if
we can make conscious the mental process through
which it has acquired its meaning, the symptom must
disappear.

The mechanism of symptom-formation differs to
some extent in the various forms of neurosis. In the
classical type of hysteria characterized by disabilities
of the motor and sensory functions of the body, such
as paralysis and anæsthesia, the psycho-analytical
account of symptom-formation necessitates a somewhat novel conception of the relation between the
cognitive and the affective aspects of mental events
and processes. Freud regards " affect " as a form of
mental energy, derived from the instincts and loosely
attached to the memory traces of ideas, which has the
attributes of a quantity that may be increased or
diminished just as a quantity of physical energy may
be increased or diminished. When such symptoms as
paralysis or motor agitation occur in hysteria, the
affect-energy pertaining to the repressed wish seems to
be deflected and converted into the innervation of the
bodily symptom ; and that is why this form of psycho-
neurosis is now known as *Conversion Hysteria*.

In another form of hysteria the capacity for
conversion seems to be lacking and the affect-energy,
compelled to remain in the mental sphere, gives rise
to morbid anxiety, with dread of some object or act

which in a normal person is not usually associated with any such feeling. This displacement of affect from one idea to another is possible because of the postulated looseness of attachment between ideas and their affects. The form of hysteria arising in this way and characterized by phobias and attacks of anxiety or dread is known as *Anxiety Hysteria.*

In anxiety hysteria the fear which conscious realization of the repressed wishes would entail is projected outwards and becomes attached to some object or situation in the outer world. These objects or situations symbolize in some way the infantile wishes, and when they are encountered they arouse in full intensity the fear that would be reasonable enough if these wishes became conscious without disguise. On the other hand, anxiety attacks can be avoided by avoiding the objects or situations that stand for the forbidden wish.

In a third type of psycho-neurosis the symptoms take the form of obsessional thoughts or compulsive acts. The patient is under some kind of compulsion to act, or think, or feel, in some particular way. He may have obsessive ideas about which he is compelled to think, or obsessive doubts or fears ; or he may feel bound to perform some particular action the triviality of which is often in striking contrast to the feeling of urgent need which forces him to do it. Here, again, it is a question of displacement of affect. The action

which is in itself so trivial symbolizes something which
is of real significance. But the compulsive act is not
as a rule, the fulfilment of an unconscious wish ; it
is rather a denial and rejection of it ; it has often the
appearance of a religious or magical rite which absolves
or protects. Such a symptom is not of the nature of
a compromise in which both the repressed and the
repressing forces are represented ; it is what is called
a *reaction-formation*, opposed to the unconscious wish,
and is derived from the repressing forces.

It is noteworthy that when the unconscious wish
tends or threatens to enter consciousness it always
gives rise to anxiety. The somatic conversion in conversion hysteria is one way of escape from anxiety,
and if the physical symptom is removed by suggestion,
as is sometimes easily done, its disappearance is often
followed by mental symptoms in the form of appre-
hensive dread or anxiety. So, also, in anxiety hysteria,
the formation of a phobia, the fastening of the displaced affect to the idea of some specific object or
situation, protects the patient from anxiety so long
as this object or situation is avoided. In the obsessional
neurosis the symptoms also prove to be means of
avoiding anxiety ; for if the patient resolutely abstains
from performing the compulsive act, or dwelling on the
obsessive thought, he is seized with unrest and
unreasonable dread.

Thus we see that in all three forms of psycho-neurosis

the formation of symptoms is a mechanism of defence against the occurrence of anxiety, just as we saw that repression is a defence against unbearable ideas or wishes. Both in repression and in symptom-formation it looks as if the Ego were trying to escape from or defend itself against something which it fears. What is it ?

THEORY OF THE LIBIDO

A T the close of our last lecture it was pointed out
that both repression and symptom formation
are ways of protecting the Ego from something too
painful to be borne. It looks, we said, as if the Ego
were afraid of something and we asked, What is it ?
The answer of psycho-analysis is that the Ego is afraid
of the Libido. This answer is fundamental in the
psycho-analytic theory of the neuroses, and we must
endeavour to understand what is meant by the terms
Ego and Libido, and how they come to stand in such
a relation to each other. In this lecture we shall examine
the theory of the Libido, and in the following lecture
we shall consider what we may call Freud's theory of
the Ego.

Libido is the term used to denote the craving for
satisfaction of the sexual instincts, just as we use the
terms hunger and thirst to denote the cravings for
satisfaction of the instincts of nutrition. It is the
driving force behind sexual activities of every kind,
and reveals itself equally in the highest manifestations
of love, in the sensual gratifications of the pervert,
and in the auto-erotic satisfactions of the child. It is
essentially a craving for pleasure of a peculiar quality
which is present in certain pleasures that are sought

51

after from infancy to old age. The theory of the Libido is thus intimately bound up with the question of the part played by pleasure in determining the behaviour of living organisms.

The part played by pleasure in the determination of human activities can only be an extension into human life of some similar principle at work in the lower animals ; and if we trace Libido-driven activities far enough back in the animal scale we may find that they can still be detected when we have reached back to a stage of phylo-genetic development in which sexual differentiation has not yet taken 'place. In other words, we may find that Libido is prior to sex, and that it is a form of the primal life energy which is only later monopolized by the sexual instincts. Moreover, it continues to manifest in the individual life after the sexual functions have apparently ceased, and is the motive force behind various interests and pursuits which have no obvious resemblance to those for which they act as substitutes.

The part played by pleasure and pain in the determination of behaviour is still a matter of controversy among psychologists and moralists, and it has become almost a commonplace with modern writers to decry as old-fashioned the view of Bentham and James Mill that pleasure and pain are the only incentives to action, and that the desire for pleasure and the avoidance of pain are the only ultimate human motives. Yet the persistence with which this view has reappeared again and again in the history of psychological and ethical speculation may lead us to suspect that it contains some sort of truth which we must accept. This theory of Psychological Hedonism affords, at first sight, a plausible explanation of human behaviour ; it is supported by much that can be found by honest introspection in our own motives, and by unprejudiced observation of the conduct of others. And yet it seems hopelessly inadequate to account for the whole of human and animal behaviour. A more satisfactory hypothesis is that which traces all our actions to instinctual impulses which are aroused by objects or circumstances specially adapted to stir them into activity. The action originating in these impulses is directed towards some end, and pleasure is an accompaniment or a consequence of the successful attainment of this end ; but a desire for pleasure is not, as a rule, or necessarily, the motive of the action. Yet it is probable that all the so-called instincts originated in pleasure-pain reactions ; or, since the laying down of the instincts must have occurred so far back in phylogenetic history that we may not be justified in ascribing consciousness of pleasure or pain to the organisms in which they arose, we must rather say that the reactions which ultimately became instinctual were those most useful for adaptation, and that in some way that we do not understand the

impulses effecting successful adaptation came to be
accompanied by pleasure as soon as mental evolution
had reached a stage at which feeling of pleasure was
possible.

But if there was from the beginning some connexion
between pleasure and the impulses effecting successful
adaptation, then it may be said that the pursuit of
pleasure was implicit in the reactions on which every
instinct is founded. We should thus find that every
instinct prompts to some form of activity, directed
towards some end, the attainment of which is accompanied by pleasure. But although each of the instincts
provides impulses towards pleasure-giving activities,
and although human conduct may be considered to
have no other ultimate source, it does not follow that
the *organism as a whole* is striving for pleasure when it
acts in obedience to one or other instinctual urge.
In human life adaptation is so complex and so difficult
of achievement that only very seldom can it be effected
by means of purely instinctual behaviour ; and in the
modifications of instinct which constitute intelligent
behaviour, the pursuit of pleasure may recede so far
into the background that it becomes indiscernible,
and conduct may diverge so far from that prescribed
by the primitive impulses that its instinctual basis
may be hard to discover.

Freud believes that our entire psychical activity
is bent upon procuring pleasure and avoiding pain,

and that it is automatically regulated by what he calls the *pleasure-principle*. But he would avoid, if possible, the teleological implications of such expressions as " striving for pleasure ", and he thinks no account of mental process is complete unless it can be stated in terms of " the distribution of quantities of mental excitation ". He roughly correlates pain, on the whole, with an excess of psychic tension, and pleasure with relaxation of tension. Pleasurable processes depend upon the mastering and discharge of the stimulus excitations which are set up in the mind, either from within or from without. One of the primary functions of the mental machine is to keep the amount of excitation as low as possible, or, at least, constant within certain limits. The striving for pleasure is thus, for Freud, a purely mechanical process," *in some way* connected with lessening, lowering, or extinguishing the amount of stimulation present in the mental apparatus," [1] and the pleasure aspect of instinctual satisfaction is the quality of feeling produced by avoidance or release of psychical tension.

The psycho-analytic theory of pleasure and pain was formulated in order to account for certain facts observed in the practice of psycho-analysis. And since the analysts' endeavours to trace neurotic symptoms to their source invariably led to repressed material related to the sexual life, it so happened that this theory

[1] Freud, *Introductory Lectures*, p. 299.

was applied more especially to the pleasure and pain associated with the satisfactions and thwartings of the sexual instincts. To what extent it is applicable to other instincts, and what these other instincts may be, is a question that was more or less put on one side for the time being ; and the main work of psycho-analysis, for many years, was to trace the sexual instinct to its source and to study its development, its vicissitudes, and its fates, as these are exemplified in, or illuminated by, the lives of neurotic patients.

The most important result of this long investigation was the formulation and gradual elaboration of the Libido-theory of the neuroses. Libido is the technical term used to indicate the energy of the sexual instincts, the force by means of which they achieve expression. At first this term was applied only to the desire or craving which presupposes an outer object towards which the libidinal impulses are directed ; but later it came to be recognized that Libido may also be turned inward or withdrawn into the Ego.

So long as we think in terms of adult sexuality the theory of the Libido and the Libido-theory of the neuroses must seem unmeaning or absurd ; but when we remember the developmental steps by which the instinct has attained its adult form, the conception of Libido is a most useful one and helps to emphasize the common element in all forms of sexual craving and gratification, whether in the normal adult, in the sexual pervert, in the sufferer from neurosis, or in the un-developed child.

I have suggested that in phylogeny Libido may be manifested prior to the appearance of sex-differentiation. In ontogenetic development, although some theoretical conclusions may be formulated con-cerning Libido-distribution in the pre-natal state, for practical purposes we need not go farther back than the time of birth. And just as in phylogeny Libido may be found prior to sex, so in the new-born babe, although sex-differentiation has been attained, the libidinal manifestations that may be observed are not located in the genital organs. We may disregard a diffuse distribution of Libido throughout the whole of the bodily tissues, especially those of the skin and the muscles, and pay attention to the most obviously libidinal activities of the new-born child. These are related to the instinctive gratification of nutritional and excretory needs. For example, unbiassed observation convinces us that a libidinal element enters into the pleasure of the infant feeding at its mother's breast. Later, this libidinal element may separate out from the nutritional act, and the child may show pleasure in the act of sucking for its own sake. Although at first sight an activity of this kind may seem far removed from sexuality, yet this oral phase of Libido-development has phylogenetic parallels which make its appearance in ontogeny explicable.

Libido-manifestations in childhood are also observed in connexion with acts of excretion. Anal activities are a source of pleasure during a certain phase of Libido-development, and at the same time an impulse to mastery, with cruel tendencies, may be very pronounced. This phase of Libido-development is of great importance in the determination of certain neurotic disorders, and the part it plays in the formation of character is one of the most astonishing discoveries of psycho-analysis. Probably no one ever encounters psycho-analytic teaching on this matter for the first time without regarding it as false and preposterous ; and yet no one who has carefully investigated a case of obsessional neurosis can ever doubt its truth.

In this so-called anal-sadistic phase of Libido-development there is still no obvious connexion with sexuality in the ordinary şense, because the Libido is not yet localized in the genital organs and the distinction of masculine and feminine does not enter into it. But the originally diffuse distribution of Libido is already giving place to some degree of that integration which, adumbrated in the phase of infantile genital organization, attains its final form in the primacy of the genital organs at puberty. Thus the Libido-function passes through a pre-genital phase, comprising two sub-phases, the oral phase and the anal-sadistic phase, in infancy, and a genital phase, characterized in childhood by the supremacy of the phallus, and reaching its final adult form at puberty.

The developmental history of the Libido, over-simplified in this description, shows a continuous progress from the originally diffuse distribution among the various impulses which form the sexual life of children, each seeking pleasure independently and having no other aim, to the final redistribution in the adult genital phase, when these impulses are re-arranged and united in the service of reproduction. But this continuous development is not always satisfactorily achieved. Any one of the libidinal impulses may be arrested in its onward progress and fail to proceed to the next phase. Such an arrest is called a *fixation*.

One of the consequences of fixation is that the volume of Libido which goes on to further development and to final organization in adult life is diminished by just that amount which is left behind at the fixation point. And since Libido-satisfaction in later life is in any case rendered hard by the restrictions imposed by culture and morality, it can easily be understood that when the forces of the love-life are weakened by previous fixation of Libido, a failure to overcome these obstacles may the more readily occur. When this happens the Libido tends to flow back towards the points of fixation and so revive desires and impulses, appropriate to an earlier phase of development, which had been to a large extent outgrown.

This turning back of Libido in the face of obstacles is technically called *regression*. A happy analogy, used by Freud, will help us to get a clear picture of the causes and the consequences of Libido-regression. He says : " If you think of a migrating people who have left large numbers at the stopping places on their way, you will see that the foremost will naturally fall back upon these positions when they are defeated or when they meet with an enemy too strong for them. And, again, the more of their number they leave behind in their progress, the sooner will they be in danger of defeat." (*Lectures*, p. 286.)

Libido-gratification in infancy has two chief characteristics : (1) it is, or tends to be, achieved without the help of any external object, i.e. it is auto-erotic, and (2) it tends to arise in connexion with the satisfying of the great organic needs—nutrition and excretion. The first object in the outer world which contributes to libidinal gratification is the mother's breast. Prompted by the need of nutrition, and probably independently of any urge towards libidinal satisfaction, the act of sucking nevertheless gives pleasure of a libidinal nature which is different from the pleasure of having the nutritional need satisfied. That this is so is shown by the fact, already referred to, that the peculiar pleasure derived from the act of sucking very soon becomes an aim in itself, irrespective of any nutritional need. And when the baby discovers that in the pursuit of this kind of pleasure its own thumb forms a satisfactory substitute for the mother's breast, the oral Libido reverts to the auto-erotism which characterizes infantile sexuality in general. In the development of the Libido the first great task for the child is to renounce auto-erotism and to find some suitable object in the outer world towards which the Libido may be directed. This is not always easy, and the varying degree of success with which it may be accomplished points to a feature of the Libido-function which probably depends upon some constitutional peculiarity the nature of which we do not know. One individual may differ from another in what is called the *adhesiveness* of the Libido, and when tenacity in holding on to a particular channel of outlet or to a particular object is excessive, it may lead to a fixation which renders normal development difficult or impossible. And, even when the normal phases of the Libido-organization are passed through without undue fixation, it is noteworthy that the love-objects of later life are apt to be modelled upon those on which the Libido first fastened in the early days of infancy. The mother's breast is the first object in the outer world to be invested with Libido, and the mother becomes the first love-object in the life of the child. The love which arises from the child's dependence on the mother who gives sustenance and protection may form the model on which all his subsequent loves are based ; or it may be that the auto-erotic object, the child's own body, becomes the prototype which cannot be departed from. When this happens the love-objects of the child's later years are those in which some resemblance to himself is seen.

The importance of the love-objects of childhood cannot be over-estimated, and when fixation on them takes place they may hold a life in thrall from child-hood to old age. All children, both male and female, take the mother as their first love-object and it might be supposed that the love which arises can be wholly accounted for by the dependent relation of the child to one who feeds and soothes and protects, and that no libidinal element enters into the love of child and parent. But it is notorious that very early in life the love of children for their parents is affected by sex-differences and that the little girl's love tends to turn quite definitely towards her father, while the love of the little boy remains fixed on his mother. By the time these love-attitudes towards the parents arise, however, repression has already begun in the mental life of the child, and he is thereby rendered ignorant of some of the libidinal aims on which his choice of a love-object is based.

This turning of the child's libidinal aims towards the parent of the opposite sex contains the germs of a child-parent relationship which, as in the myth of King Oedipus, would lead a son to murder his father and marry his mother ; it affords the first indications of that probably innate tendency towards incest against which stringent taboos or laws have had to be set up in every part of the world and in every age.

In the normal course of Libido-development the Oedipus relation is in time outgrown. It may be passed through, as any other phase of development is passed through, and die down and disappear when the next phase is due. But here, as in the course of Libido-organization, normal development may be arrested by fixation, and instead of the decay or destruction of the Oedipus complex, there occurs only its repression. When this happens the incestuous attitude implicit in the Oedipus situation will persist in the unconscious and may express itself later in some form of neurosis.

Thus we see that there may be fixation of the Libido at any of the stages passed through on the way to its adult organization, and there may be fixation upon early love-objects or types of object-choice. And when the Libido turns back, in the face of obstacles to its satisfaction, the regression may be towards one or other or both of these forms of fixation.

The importance of fixation and regression will be more easily appreciated when we study the Libido-theory of the neuroses. People who fall ill of a neurosis do so because the possibility of satisfaction of the Libido has in some way been denied to them. Their illness is a result of *privation*. But it does not follow that every person who suffers privation must necessarily succumb to neurosis. Other factors must be present, and much will depend on the nature of the privation and on the character of the person who suffers it. In people who do not develop a neurosis in consequence of privation there would seem to be a mobility and plasticity of the Libido instead of the adhesiveness which leads to fixation. In virtue of such mobility, if one form of satisfaction is denied another may take its place ; if one object has to be abandoned another may be substituted for it. The most important form of substitution is that known as *sublimation*, in which the sexual aim of an impulse is abandoned and the Libido is directed to the attainment of some other goal. This new aim is genetically related to the sexual aim, but is socially more acceptable and also, perhaps, socially more valuable. Such a substitution is called sublimation in conformity to the ethical standard which ranks social ends higher than personal or selfish ends.

Some individuals have a much greater capacity for sublimation than others, and can bear privation of libidinal satisfaction without falling ill. But sublimation can never carry off more than a certain proportion of Libido, and although these people may escape a definite neurosis they are often unhappy and dissatisfied, or they display various eccentricities of character and conduct. Only when deveolpment of the Libido has been faulty and the amount available for adult life has been diminished by extensive fixations in childhood does privation lead to neurosis. For when privation occurs these early fixations on infantile forms of gratification, or on infantile love-objects, are reanimated by the regressive flow of the Libido, and thus reinforced would seek satisfaction and lead to issue in action were it not for the censorship and inhibitions exerted by the Ego.

But regression of the Libido to the points of fixation does not take place directly ; there is an intermediate phase in which the old pathways are opened up. When in the development of the Libido the pleasures obtained from infantile activities have to be renounced, the channels and objects through which such pleasures are gained are not wholly relinquished by the Libido. They retain enough Libido-energy to give rise to phantasy, although not enough to urge to gratification in actuality. The renunciation of pleasure is not easily accomplished unless some compensation can be found, and the mental activity of phantasy, in which what once was actual is now enjoyed merely in imagination, has ever been man's most ready recompense for lost joys. When the libidinal satisfactions of childhood have to give way to the necessities of the actual world, to the claims of culture and morality, they may still be tolerated in phantasy, so long as their unreal

F

nature is recognized and no impulse to make them actual arises. But when privation in the sphere of permissible Libido-outlets is experienced, when the Libido turns back in face of obstacles arising from without or from within, the phantasies form its first line of retreat. *Introversion* of the Libido occurs, and the fresh access of energy thus conveyed to the phantasies causes so much tension that they press towards realization in actuality. Now, however, they meet the full weight of the repressing forces, mental conflict ensues, the phantasies are repressed, and the Libido retreats to the fixation-point in the unconscious on which the phantasies were based.

The part played by phantasy in the production of neurosis has proved far greater than was at first supposed. In the course of analysis the symptoms can be traced back to their origin in experiences of childhood which are strongly charged with Libido ; but it is often found that the experiences related have never been actual experiences at all. They are merely phantasies which have been repressed. It may be thought that such products of the imagination cannot have any causal connexion with the formation of neurotic symptoms ; but the contrary is true. Although phantasies have no material reality they have psychical reality, and in the field of the neuroses psychical reality is all-important.

Our knowledge of those features of the Libido which

have been referred to so far was derived from the psycho-analytic investigation of the psycho-neuroses— hysteria and obsessional neurosis. The cure of disease was the original aim of these investigations, and a gratifying amount of success was achieved in relieving conditions that were amenable to no other method of treatment. It was disappointing therefore to find that in another group of related disorders, the psychoses or true insanities, such as dementia præcox and paranoia, no therapeutic effect could be obtained. This failure seemed to show that the Libido-theory of the neuroses did not apply to these graver conditions and that consequently the psycho-analytic method could teach us nothing about their causes or their cure.

Yet in one particular at least there seemed to be a complete parallel between the two groups. In both it appeared that there was a withdrawal of Libido from objects in the outer world, in both the capacity for love was diminished or lost. But analysis showed that in hysteria and obsessional neurosis, although the Libido was withdrawn from external objects, object- love was still held on to in the phantasies ; whilst in dementia præcox and other psychoses no such dis- position of the Libido could be found. Corresponding to this difference was the fact that in the analysis of hysteria and obsessional neurosis the retention of the capacity for love was manifested in the phenomenon of *transference*, in which feelings of love or hate became detached from the love-objects of the phantasies and transferred to the person of the analyst. The Libido could thus be located throughout the course of the illness. When withdrawn from objects in the outer world it turned inwards to those of the phantasies, and in the course of analysis it turned outwards again to the physician.

From the analysts' point of view, the problem presented by dementia præcox was : What happens to the Libido when it is withdrawn from objects in the outer world ?   A characteristic trait in dementia præcox behaviour points the way to the solution. The sufferer from this disorder has delusions of greatness which remind us of similar traits in children and primitive peoples, e.g. belief in the omnipotence of thought and in the power of magical words and gestures. In dementia præcox it would seem that the Libido withdrawn or forced from the outer world has returned to the Ego and that the investment of the Ego by excess of Libido is the cause of the megalomania.

The realization that in dementia præcox the Libido withdrawn from objects becomes concentrated on the Ego marked an important stage in the development of the Libido-theory. In the original use of the term, Libido was confined to what we now refer to as object-Libido, that is to say Libido directed towards objects in the outer world. The new conception was that Libido can be directed towards the self ; and to this disposition of the Libido the term *narcissism* was applied. Freud supposed that narcissism is the original infantile state, and that object-love is a later development. The primary auto-erotic tendencies of infancy are an indication of this original direction of Libido towards the bodily self, but we cannot rightly speak of Ego-Libido until something that can be called an Ego has arisen ; and, as we shall see in a subsequent lecture, the growth of the Ego is a gradual process.

At one time Freud believed the Ego to be the original reservoir of the Libido from which it overflowed on to objects. He conceived the relation of Ego-Libido to object-Libido in a way which he illustrated by an analogy taken from the observation of primitive organisms. He said : " Think of the simplest forms of life consisting of a little mass of only slightly differentiated protoplasmic substances. They extend protrusions which are called pseudopodia into which the protoplasm overflows. They can, however, again withdraw these extensions of themselves and reform themselves into a mass. We compare this extending of protrusions to the radiation of Libido on to the objects, while the greatest volume of Libido may yet remain within the Ego ; we infer that under normal conditions Ego-Libido can transform itself into object-Libido without difficulty and that this can again subsequently be absorbed into the Ego." [1] As we shall see, Freud in some of his later writings has considerably modified this view.

[1] Freud, *Introductory Lectures*, p. 347.

By means of this conception, however, he undertook to describe in terms of the Libido-theory some conditions of normal life, such as the state of the mind in sleep, in organic illness, and in the condition of " being in love ". In sleep all Libido is withdrawn from objects and a state of complete narcissism ensues. In organic illness Libido is also largely withdrawn from objects and concentrated on the affected part of the body. A person suffering severe pain loses interest in things and ceases to love. In the condition of being in love the Ego-Libido gets poured out towards the loved person ; the Ego is depleted of Libido and, in consequence, the lover feels humble and unworthy whilst the loved person is over-estimated and idealized.

The conception of Ego-Libido introduces an important distinction between the libidinal and the egoistic aspects of the self. Freud distinguishes narcissism from egoism and says that narcissism is the libidinal complement of egoism. He speaks of egoism when it is a question of non-libidinal interests ; narcissism implies the satisfaction of libidinal needs. Thus the distinction between interest and Libido corresponds to the distinction, so often invoked, between Ego-instincts and sexual instincts.

Belief that accumulation of Libido in the Ego is the normal condition of infancy is supported by the occurrence of narcissism as a perversion, by the observable auto-erotism of children, and by the megalomanic traits in the mentality of children and savages ; and the narcissism of the psychoses appears as a secondary narcissism due to an influx of regressive Libido reanimating the primary narcissism of infancy.

The distribution of the Libido between Ego and objects is a very variable one. Some people are more narcissistic than others ; but in everyone there remains a certain amount of the original narcissism of childhood, and this may become augmented to a degree that makes a normal life impossible. In infancy autoerotic activities are the only outlet for the Libido until an object in the outer world is found. Contact with the world external to the body provides the opportunity for the turning of the Libido outwards, away from the self ; but the need for such direction of the Libido towards outer objects is probably implicit in its very nature. Just as a monocellular organism, when it grows to a certain size, must divide into two or perish, so, Libido confined to the self must find some outlet to the external world when its volume exceeds a certain amount which may vary in different individuals. For everyone there is a limit to the quantity of Ego-Libido that is compatible with health. Thus from the beginning a turning of Libido outwards and its attachment to real objects outside the self is a necessity for healthy life, and " in the last resort we must begin to love in order that we may not fall ill, and must fall ill if, in consequence of frustration, we cannot love ".[1]

[1] Freud, *Collected Papers*, vol. iv, p. 42.

THE EGO IN FREUDIAN PSYCHOLOGY

IN the early days of psycho-analysis it came to be realized that in searching for the origin and meaning of symptoms the analyst was tracing the history of the patient's Libido, discovering at what points in its development it had gone astray, and to what objects it had become attached when it was withdrawn from application in the outer world. Resistance to the recall of repressed memories was recognized from the beginning, and the forces that caused the resistance were identified with those that had originally caused the repression. These two sets of forces seemed to be concerned in all the mental processes which the analyst had to study. On the one hand were all those impulses and desires which have behind them the driving force of the Libido; on the other hand were all those forces, whatever they might be, which are opposed to Libido-strivings and lead to repression. Since the final goal of Libido-striving is race-preservation, the repressing forces were identified with those underlying the biological antithesis of race-preservation, namely self-preservation; and the forces ministering to self-preservation were given the name of Ego-instincts in opposition to the sexual instincts which are the carriers of the forces of the Libido.

It is obvious that the term Ego-instincts needs defining more precisely before it can be usefully employed ; and, indeed, each of its component parts needs defining before we can understand all that psycho-analysts include under the term Ego-instincts. That is to say, we must know what is meant by Ego, and we must know what is meant by instincts, before we can know what is meant by Ego-instincts. In his earlier writings Freud was content to leave vague and undefined many of the terms he was compelled to use. In recording his observations and discoveries he was, to some extent, obliged to use traditional forms of expression, for he was unwilling to define terms or to describe in detail any mental process until the things denoted or connoted by the term, or the mental process to be described, had been subjected to elucidation in actual analysis. Thus, while we find him defining with precision the terms he used in his description of the development of the sexual instincts, and going into elaborate detail when he tells us about the vicissitudes and fates of the Libido, he was for many years unable or unwilling to say much about those Ego-instincts to which he ascribed the repressing forces. Yet on practical grounds this indefiniteness was perhaps justifiable, and on theoretical grounds it was explicable. For analysis of the psycho-neuroses could often be carried to a satisfactory conclusion without any serious question arising about the source of the

Ego-instincts, and without any clue to their nature and mode of functioning being afforded. Indeed, it appeared that just as our knowledge of the early organizations and dispositions of the Libido, and of the way the sexual instinct acquires its final form, was arrived at by investigating those forms of neurosis in the causation of which disturbances of Libido-development was the main factor; so, analytical knowledge of the constitution and dynamics of the Ego must be obtained through the examination of disorders in which are to be found disturbances and disintegrations of the Ego itself; that is to say, by the analytic investigation of the true psychoses such as dementia præcox and paranoia.

The application to these disorders of the principles derived from the psycho-analytic study of the psycho-neuroses was hardly possible until the conception of Ego-Libido and narcissism was formulated. It then became evident that the lack of success in the analytic investigation and treatment of the psychoses was in some measure due to the absence of transference, owing to narcissistic fixation of the Libido; and it seemed that some modification of technique would have to be introduced before any great progress in this direction could be obtained. Up to the present time not much advance in this respect has been achieved, but, nevertheless, a beginning has been made and various important mechanisms underlying psychotic disorders have been discovered. Perhaps the most noteworthy results of these investigations so far are those pertaining to the analysis of the Ego, but much work on this subject must yet be done before our analytical knowledge of the Ego and its developmental history can be compared with what we have learnt about the Libido.

Thus we see that the psycho-analytic theory of the Ego, in so far as it has been formulated, is of relatively recent appearance in the literature of Psycho-analysis. In former days the Ego was sometimes referred to as being the source of the repressing forces in the neuroses and of the censorship of dreams; but the conflict between the opposing forces from which both neurotic symptoms and dreams resulted, was not usually depicted as a struggle between Ego and Libido, but rather as a struggle between the preconscious and the unconscious systems of the mind. What may be called the discovery of the unconscious was the first great achievement of psycho-analysis—not so much a discovery of its existence, for its existence, in some form, had been admitted by many former workers; but a discovery of its nature, of its content, and of the laws and modes of its functioning.

Much of our knowledge of the unconscious was gained by the application of the psycho-analytic method to the interpretation of dreams, and in his great work on this subject Freud laid the foundations of those theories of the dynamics of mental life which will always be associated with his name. Concurring in the view of Fechner that dreams arise in some region of the mind other than that concerned in waking thought, he compared the apparatus of the mind to a compound instrument, such as a microscope, in which there are fanciful locations or regions that form no tangible part of the apparatus. The component parts of the psychic apparatus he called systems, and these systems he regarded as having a constant spatial or topographical relation to each other. In this way he introduced the idea of psychic locality or mental topography into his description of mental process, and he has continued to make use of this notion up to the present time.

Since all mental activity is supposed to be based upon the model of the reflex arc, the psychic apparatus is described as being provided with a sensory or perceptual end and a motor end. The function of such a mental apparatus is to discharge through the motor end any stimulus that may enter at the sensory end. This is its sole function. The state of excitation produced by stimulus is felt as discomfort, and the relief or gratification accompanying discharge of stimulus is felt as pleasure. Such an elementary psychic system is dominated by the pleasure-principle, and the pursuit of pleasure may be said to be its sole aim.

But this description of an elementary psychic

apparatus is an abstraction, and it is doubtful if, even in the most lowly organisms, anything approaching this simplicity of arrangement is ever found. For every living creature exists in an environment which compels some modification of the pleasure-principle if the organism is to continue to live. The nature of this modification can be studied in the life-history of the human infant.

Before it is born a child has no unsatisfied wishes : all its wants are provided for in a world that exists solely for its enjoyment ; but in the process of being born this state of bliss is rudely interrupted and a terrifying experience is undergone. The unborn babe becomes the sport of forces which it is utterly helpless to resist, the Nirvana-like peace of its life is taken from it, and, if it is capable of feeling any emotion at all, fear and anxiety must arise. Separated from its mother, the need of air becomes insistent, and it is compelled to exert itself in breathing. The world into which it has come is cold, compared with the warmth of the mother's body, and in response to this fresh stimulus it has " no language but a cry ". But if it is ministered to, protected from cold, and if its breathing is unimpeded, it will cease crying and will fall asleep. For the time being it has got back to something approaching the conditions of its life before it was born. But soon a new need arises. Outer coverings can replace the womb as a protection from cold, the act of breathing can supply the oxygen formerly obtained from the maternal blood, but the nutritive material derived from the same source is now lacking. Hunger sets in, and here again the helpless infant can do nothing but cry. When it is fed and this want satisfied it again relapses into sleep.

We can imagine the child at this stage to be endowed with a primitive mental apparatus such as has been described, and from other researches we know that one of the chief characteristics of such a mental system is the freedom of movement of the excitations set up by stimuli at the receptive end of the mental arc. They move freely in all directions, seeking an outlet for discharge which will secure satisfaction and bring the system to rest again. The excitations provided by hunger may move towards the motor end of the arc, but there are as yet no paths to motor activity adequate to the situation ; and the movements set up in the mental apparatus therefore pass backwards to the sensory end of the arc and revive with hallucinatory vividness the sensations experienced, on some former occasion, when the child was being fed. The hallucinatory revival of these sensations, brought about by regression of the stimulus-excitations to the sensory end of the mental arc, brings a temporary satisfaction ; but when, as with hunger, the need giving rise to the stimulus is not really satisfied, the movement within the mental apparatus is set up again very soon. Experience reveals the inadequacy of regression and a secondary system arises within the mind which has as its function the inhibition of the tendency to regression and the direction of the impulses towards the motor end of the arc. Behaviour must be such that the outer world is acted upon and so changed that a real gratification is wrested from it in place of the illusory gratification of phantasy.

The secondary mental system thus arising is said to be actuated by the *reality-principle* in contrast to the *pleasure-principle* which dominates the primary system. At first the secondary system acts solely in the service of the primary system. It tries to ensure that the satisfactions sought by the primary system are obtained as real satisfactions, and to learn the lesson that the obstacles in the way, and the pain that may be encountered, are part of the nature of things which has to be recognized and if possible circumvented. But there comes a time in the course of mental development when the things that give pleasure to the primary system give pain or discomfort to the secondary system. This change marks an important stage in the development of personality, for it forms the basis of repression and the beginnings of the two mental systems which we call the unconscious and the preconscious. The primary system is the forerunner of the unconscious system, and all that is characteristic of the primary system can be recognized in the nature of the unconscious. So, also, the secondary system becomes the preconscious system, and is closely bound up with those functions commonly ascribed to consciousness, such as reason, foresight, and the sense of values.

We are here coming near to something like a rudimentary conception of the Ego, and when we remember that the content of the unconscious, in so far as the unconscious is a result of repression, is pre-eminently composed of libidinal impulses or wishes, we may see that the original opposition between the primary and secondary systems is the forerunner of the opposition which has been postulated as existing between the Ego and the Libido. We have, indeed, a series of oppositions which have successively been brought to light in the development of psycho-analytic theory ; primary system versus secondary system, pleasure principle versus reality principle, unconscious system versus preconscious system ; and there would seem to be some factor common to them all which perhaps finds its fullest expression in the formula : Libido versus Ego.

Before going on to consider Freud's views on the nature of the Ego, it is necessary to ask if there is any difference between the Ego of Psycho-analysis and the Ego described by writers on General Psychology. We may disregard, for the moment, the question of "The Pure Ego", sometimes discussed by psychologists, and compare the Freudian Ego with the empirical Ego of general psychology. When we do so it would seem that, in sharply separating the Libido from the Ego, Freud is, in fact, splitting the empirical Ego into two parts, one of which he sets up in opposition to the other under the name of the Libido. In all descriptions of the self, bodily appetites and instincts, and the activities to which they give rise, have hitherto been included among the constituents of the Ego. The empirical Ego has been described as comprising all that a man can call " his ", and a man must call his instincts his, however much he may disapprove of or reject them. As Freud himself has said, " we are warned not to forget that the Libido of a given person is fundamentally part of that person and cannot be contrasted with him as if it were something external." [1]

It may be contended that in states of dissociated personality a man might disown the impulses of the secondary self, and in the same way it may be held that the libidinal wishes that are repressed form no part of the constitution of the Ego. But even if this be conceded it would imply only a distinction between the Ego and the repressed, not a distinction between Ego and Libido ; for not all libidinal impulses are repressed, and those that are unrepressed would still form part of the Ego. The opposition of the Ego to the repressed Libido is, indeed, the foundation of the conflict, which leads to neurosis, but it would seem to be subversive

[1] Freud, *Introductory Lectures*, p. 338.

of psycho-analytic doctrine to include unrepressed (i.e. ego-syntonic) object-libido among the constituents of the Ego. Thus, it would seem, we cannot identify the Ego of psycho-analysis with the empirical Ego of academic psychology, and in using the term Ego in the exposition of Freud's views we must do so only in the sense in which it is used by him.

Until comparatively recently Freud made little use of the term Ego in his writings, except for the somewhat vague references to the Ego-instincts which he opposed to the sexual instincts in dealing with the subject of repression. His early researches brought out so forcibly the enormous part played by the sexual instincts in mental life that for practical purposes he made a division by dichotomy of instinctive processes into sexual and non-sexual; and those that are non-sexual he called Ego-instincts.

At first the Ego was spoken of as if it were conterminous with the conscious and preconscious system of the mind. It was regarded as a coherent organization of mental processes, bound up with consciousness, which controlled the thoughts and actions of everyday life, rejected those that were unacceptable, went to sleep at night, and even then maintained the censorship of dreams. It was in practice identified with the conscious personality. But in carrying out analyses it became clear that, if the Ego is the source of the repressing forces, then part of the Ego itself must be unconscious. For when the resistances are investigated it is often found that the motive for resistance is unconscious, and behaves like other unconscious material in that, without becoming conscious, it produces powerful effects. The unconscious part of the Ego is not latent in the sense in which the preconscious is latent, for it requires special work in order to make it conscious.

But although part of the Ego is unconscious we must start our investigation from the side of consciousness. And here we may call to mind Freud's division of the mental apparatus into systems. The most important of these are the unconscious and the preconscious. The preconscious is closely related to consciousness, inasmuch as its content may readily become conscious ; it is " accessible ", as Dr. Broad would say. Consciousness itself is, to begin with, bound up with perception. Freud refers it to the surface of the mental apparatus which he calls the system of Perceptual Consciousness—a system which, in his topographical scheme, he places on the boundary between outer and inner, enveloping the other psychic systems and facing towards the outer world. He thinks only that can become conscious which was, at some time, conscious perception.

But not all that is conscious comes from outer perception. By inner perception we experience feelings and emotions which originate in the deepest strata of the mind. These, when not under repression, become conscious directly without the intermediary of preconscious connecting links ; but the residues of conscious perception which enter into thought processes—the memories of concrete things and their relations—cannot become conscious without first becoming linked up with preconscious intermediaries. From a consideration of certain peculiarities of speech observable in dementia præcox, Freud has come to the conclusion that these preconscious intermediaries consist of the memory-residues of words ; and pre-eminently of words heard, since all our knowledge of words is derived primarily from auditory perceptions. The difference, he says, between an unconscious idea and a conscious or preconscious idea is that in the latter the memory of the concrete thing and its relations has joined up with the memory of the corresponding words. Using Dr. Broad's term, we may say that what makes a thought accessible is the possibility of putting it into words. Freud does not forget the type of thinker whose memories of both words and things are predominantly visual, but he maintains that relations, which are the peculiar characteristic of thought, cannot be expressed visually.

It is interesting to note that this view of the relation of the unconscious to the conscious, which was put forward by Freud in 1915, reappears in the writings of Professor Watson, the Behaviourist, as if it were a discovery of his own, and one very damaging to the Freudian conception of the unconscious. In an article on Behaviourism contributed to the current number of the official organ of this Institute, the *Journal of Philosophical Studies*,[1] Professor Watson says : " Freud's realm of the unconscious thus turns out to be a natural science realm—that of the unverbalized." Compare this with Freud's statement : " The conscious idea comprises the concrete idea plus the verbal idea corresponding to it, whilst the unconscious idea is that of the thing alone." [2] Were it not that Professor Watson has told us that he has no belief in the existence of any ideas, either conscious or unconscious, we might suppose that these two statements mean the same thing.

The perceptual system, which includes the pre-conscious, and through which we come to know the outer world and our inner thoughts and feelings is the nucleus of the Ego. It is through its origin in the perceptual system that the Ego becomes bound up with consciousness. But, as we have seen, part of the Ego is unconscious, so that the antithesis of Ego and Unconscious cannot be maintained. In view of the many contradictions and confusions which retention of his earlier terminology seemed to entail, Freud, when he came to investigate the constitution of the Ego, introduced an entirely new set of terms into his account of the structure and

[1] Vol. i, No. 4, p. 464.
[2] Freud, *Collected Papers*, vol. iv, p. 134.

working of the mind. He regards all the differentia-
tions within the individual mind as having arisen
from an elementary unconscious psychic mass which
he calls *das Es*—a term already used by Nietzsche
(and by Groddeck) in a somewhat similar sense. (By
English psycho-analysts *das Es* is being rendered
as *the Id*.) An individual is a psychic Id out of which
is developed the Ego, the nucleus of which is formed
by the perceptual system. If we try to represent it
graphically the Id will not be depicted as being
entirely enveloped by the Ego, but only to the extent
of the surface formed by the perceptual system. Nor
is the Ego sharply separated from the Id, but blends
with it below. Part of the Id, namely the repressed
material, is separated from the Ego by the barrier
of the resistances which maintain the repression,
but the repressed can find a pathway to the Ego
through that part of the Id which, though unconscious,
is not repressed.

The Ego is really a part of the Id which has been
modified by the influence of the outer world, brought
to bear upon it through the system of perceptual
consciousness. The contact with reality thus effected
compels the Ego to adopt the reality-principle and to
abandon the pleasure-principle which holds absolute
sway in the Id. Moreover, the Ego tries to bring
the influence of the outer world to bear upon the Id
and its purposes ; it stands for reason and circum-

spection, prudence and discretion, in contradistinction to the Id which contains the passions.

The opposition between the Ego and the Id is at first merely an opposition brought about by the need for making the pleasure-principle subservient to the reality-principle in the interests of adaptation. The Ego as the agent of the reality-principle endeavours to guide and direct the libidinal impulses of the Id, and there is at first no necessary incompatibility between the aims of the Id and the aims of the Ego. But just as the history of the Libido shows that it comes to its final form through a series of successive changes, so also there is a development of the Ego which may or may not keep pace with the corresponding changes in the growth of the Libido.

The most important change in the development of the Ego is the occurrence of a differentiation within the Ego itself, whereby a criticising faculty arises, opposed to the complaisant Ego which too readily adopts as its own the aims of the Id. This is the change which has already been referred to in our description of the primary and secondary systems of the mental apparatus, where we said that in the course of mental development a time comes when that which gives pleasure to the primary system gives pain to the secondary system. We now come to Freud's account of what the change is. It is the development of a differentiated portion of the Ego which he calls the

Ego-ideal or *super-Ego* ; the Ego-ideal is the source of the moral conscience, of self-observation and self-criticism, of the forces of repression and the censorship of dreams.

The analysis of the Ego has already led to some important conclusions concerning the origin and significance of that side of the mind to which is commonly attributed the " higher nature " of man. The need for the formation of an Ego-ideal—an ideal of what the Ego would like to be—arises from the wounds to childhood's narcissism which increasing contact with the actual world entails. The child who in the days of infancy had felt himself to be omnipotent comes to know himself as weak and powerless ; his magic words and gestures effect no real changes in his world ; all the infantile perfections which had gratified his self-love become the objects of criticism and admonition from his elders, and a dawning sense of his own unworthiness completes the overthrow of his early narcissism. But this frustration of his self-love is a privation which he cannot endure ; he sets up within his Ego an ideal of what he would like to be, and this ideal he can love as he loved his real Ego when he was his own ideal. But self-love cannot now be gratified unless the Ego lives up to the standard imposed by the Ego-ideal, and to ensure this gratification a " conscience " must arise which watches the Ego and imposes upon it the demands of the Ego-ideal.

Freud sometimes speaks of conscience as if it were a special institution in the mind, distinct from both the Ego and the Ego-ideal; but his account of how the Ego-ideal arises is in keeping with his definite inclusion of conscience as one of its functions. In the delusions of being watched, so common in certain mental disorders, the roots from which conscience has grown are laid bare. Sufferers from this affliction complain that all their thoughts and actions are being watched and commented upon; they hear voices which describe or criticize all they think or do. These voices are the representatives of the parental and social criticisms which first wounded the infantile narcissism and prompted the setting up of an Ego-ideal.

The origin of the Ego-ideal and the occasion of its formation are to be found, like so much else that psycho-analysis has taught us, in the child-parent relationship of the Oedipus situation. Before the love-attachments of the Oedipus situation arise, however, an earlier form of emotional tie between child and parent is found. A small boy takes his father as his ideal; he wants to be like him and to do as he does. As may often be observed in his play, he identifies himself with his father. *Identification* is quite distinct from a libidinal tie such as that which a little later arises between the small boy and his mother. He would like to *be* his father; he would like to *have* his mother. Identification is an earlier form of emotional tie than libidinal attachment, and under certain circumstances object-love may regress to identification.

A love-object that has been lost or renounced may be re-established within the Ego by means of identification. This is what happens in melancholia. The melancholiac's self-condemnation is really hostility towards someone that has been loved and lost, expressed as condemnation of the Ego which has identified itself with the lost love-object.

The process of identification is of frequent occurrence, especially in the early phases of mental development, and Freud suggests that the character of the Ego is very largely a result of identifications with love-objects that have been lost or have had to be renounced. He says that in women who have had many love-experiences in their lives, it is easy to discover in their characters the traits due to identifications with the lovers whom they have lost or abandoned. He even thinks that if identifications become too numerous, too strong, and mutually incompatible, they may lead to a disintegration of the Ego such as is seen in cases of multiple personality. Individuals vary in the amount of resistance they offer to such moulding of their characters by means of identification, and the consequences of such identifications in later life may be slight and evanescent ; but the effects of the first identifications of all—those occurring in early childhood—are strong and lasting.

Identifications with the parents form the nucleus of the Ego-ideal, and the formation of the Ego-ideal is the outcome of that phase of sexual development which is dominated by the Oedipus relationship between child and parent ; indeed its formation is primarily brought about by the need for mastering and repressing the Oedipus complex. The parents are the obstacles in the way of realization of Oedipus desires, and the infantile Ego gets strength to overcome these desires by setting up within itself the same obstructions and prohibitions by means of identification with the parents. Their point of view is, as it were, adopted by the Ego, but the modification of the Ego thus arising remains isolated and confronts the rest of the content of the Ego as the Ego-ideal or super-Ego. As time goes on the Ego-ideal thus formed is reinforced by later identifications and by the precepts and example of all those who play the part of parent-substitutes in the individual's life. In this way, according to Freud, conscience is formed, and any discrepancy between the Ego's performance and the claims of conscience gives rise to a sense of guilt.

Identification is an unconscious process and the Ego-ideal formed by identification is largely unconscious also. The criticizing function of the Ego-ideal may be unconsciously performed, so that a patient may suffer from an intense sense of guilt without being able to say what he is guilty of ; and, further, the sense of guilt may itself be unconscious, so that the patient does not feel guilty, but ill. Analysis shows that the illness is a form of self-punishment for guilty wishes of which the Ego knows nothing. Here the Ego-ideal knows more than the Ego about the unconscious Id.

The Ego-ideal is the heir of the Oedipus complex, from which it derives its power ; and by setting up its ideal the Ego masters the Oedipus complex, but in doing so it subordinates itself in some degree to the Id. The Ego-ideal, owing to its derivation from the Oedipus complex, represents the inner psychic world, as opposed to the outer " real " world, which led to the formation of the Ego. To the Id the Ego is the representative of the outer world ; to the Ego the Ego-ideal is the representative of the Id.

The Ego-ideal is largely a reaction-formation against the libidinal impulses of the Id, and it assists the Ego in its task of trying to overcome the Id, which is entirely non-moral, and consequently a source of danger to the Ego. But just because it is a reaction-formation there is a danger that it may become over-moral and cruel in its severity towards the Ego. We thus get a picture of the Ego assailed on three sides, in bondage to three different masters each of whom it must satisfy if it is to be free from anxiety. Danger to the Ego may come from the outside world, from the libido of the Id, or from the severity of the Ego-ideal.

It is not always easy to translate the accepted doctrines of psycho-analysis into the new terminology which has accompanied Freud's division of the mind into the Id, the Ego, and the Ego-ideal. And this difficulty is accentuated by the fact that, coincidently with his adoption of this tri-partite division, he has had occasion to modify some parts of his former teaching. For example, when he first propounded his conception of narcissism he held that the Ego was the original reservoir of the Libido, and that from the Ego the Libido overflowed towards objects very much as an amœboid organism may push out protoplasmic feelers towards the outer world. We have now to recognize, however, that when the distinction between Ego and Id has arisen, the Id is the great reservoir of Libido. At first all Libido is accumulated in the Id, but is directed towards the Ego (*primary narcissism*), whilst the Ego is still inchoate and feeble. Erotic impulses arise in the Id as urgent needs, and the investment of objects with Libido emanates from the Id. The Ego comes to know of these libidinal impulses, directed towards objects, and either accepts them or tries to defend itself against them by repression. Or, if it cannot accept them, the Ego may more effectually master the Id by identifying itself with the object that has to be renounced. In so doing it tries to impose itself upon the

Id as a substitute for the lost love-object : it is as if it said : " Look, you can love me, too, I am so like the object you loved ! " The narcissism thus produced by identification is therefore a *secondary narcissism*, due to an influx to the Ego of Libido which has been withdrawn from objects.

Such withdrawal of Libido from objects and the turning of it on to the Ego involves a renunciation of libidinal aims, a desexualization of Libido, which is a sort of sublimation. Indeed, Freud thinks it possible that all sublimation may be effected in this way ; that is to say, by the Ego converting object-Libido into narcissistic Libido in order thereafter to set before it another aim.

Let me summarize briefly the more important points in Freud's conception of the Ego. The mind in its beginning is conceived as an unconscious Id. The Ego arises as a modification of the Id, produced by contact with the outer world through the perceptual system. It comes into existence in response to the claims of reality, and for the purpose of securing a real satis-faction of the impulses of the Id, which disregards reality and is dominated by the pleasure-principle. By means of identification with the parents or one of the parents, an Ego-ideal is set up within the Ego, and, as a super-Ego, adopts the critical and condemnatory attitude of the parents towards the libidinal impulses of the Id. The Ego-ideal functions as conscience, and is the instigator of the repressions effected by the Ego.

Besides the early identifications which enter into the formation of the Ego-ideal, other identifications take place throughout life, and Freud thinks the character of the Ego is largely a result of identifications with love-objects that have been lost or renounced.

There is little in this account of the constitution and functions of the Ego that corresponds to anything we ordinarily call instinct, and we must postpone consideration of the so-called Ego-instincts until we have considered the problem of instinct as a whole. This we shall do in our next lecture.

THEORY OF THE INSTINCTS

IN our last lecture we were occupied with some of the conclusions at which Freud had arrived in the course of his analytic investigation of the Ego, but we failed to find any functions or activities of the Ego described by him which could be classed along with those ordinarily spoken of as instincts. We, therefore, left open the question of what we are to understand by Ego-instincts, until we had considered more fully the problem of instinct as a whole, and more especially until we had discovered what meaning should be attached to this term in Freudian psychology. For the word instinct has been used by psychologists in so many different senses that it is necessary for us to make sure what any particular writer includes under this term.

There is probably no department of psychology at the present time which exhibits so many varieties of opinion as does this topic of instinct or the instincts. On the one hand we have the Behaviourists, and others of similar ways of thinking, who deny that there is any such thing as instinct at all ; who would explain all forms of animal and human behaviour in terms of reflex action, and would relegate to the category of conditioned reflexes all that is usually called instinct. On the other hand, among those who admit the existence of instincts, we find great diversity of opinion concerning the kinds of experience that should be referred to as instinctive or instinctual. Some writers regard as instinctive every form of co-ordinated bodily movement which needs little or no practice for its accurate execution, the co-ordination being innately determined. Others restrict the instincts to purposive actions which are accurately performed without any previous experience or learning. Others, again, confine the term to the impulses towards satisfaction of fundamental needs of the organism, such as self-preservation and reproduction.

One of the most noteworthy contributions to the problems of instinct, in recent years, is that which is found in the writings of Professor McDougall, and the sense in which he uses the term is perhaps that in which it is used by the majority of psychologists in this country. He defines an instinct as " an innate disposition which determines the organism to perceive (to pay attention to) any object of a certain class, and to experience in its presence a certain emotional excitement and an impulse to action which finds expression in a specific mode of behaviour in relation to that object ".[1] That is to say, all instinctual activity has three sides : a sensory or perceptual side, an emotional or affective side, and a motor or executive

[1] W. McDougall, *An Outline of Psychology*, p. 110.

side. Some object is perceived or some situation arises
which excites the instinct-disposition, and this excitement is accompanied by some specific emotion and by
a felt impulse to act in some specific way. The specific
form of behaviour is sometimes regarded as the
essential part, but the accompanying emotional
experience is inseparably connected with the problem
of instinct. Dr. McDougall describes fourteen human
instincts, the activity of each of which is accompanied
by a specific form of emotional excitement.   For
example, the instinct of escape or flight is accompanied
by the emotion of fear, the instinct of combat by the
emotion of anger, the instinct of repulsion by the
emotion of disgust. But it is by its motor expression,
by the goal towards which behaviour tends, that
he defines an instinct. For Mr. Shand, on the other
hand, the problems of behaviour have their centre in
the emotions. What Dr. McDougall describes as the
typical instincts, Mr. Shand calls " emotional
dispositions ", and he confines the term instinct to
the innately organized motor mechanisms through
which the emotional dispositions achieve their end.
Dr. McDougall regards such motor mechanisms not
as instincts, but as merely the instruments of the
instincts, for any one instinctive impulse may make
use of a variety of motor mechanisms.

In a somewhat similar way, however, we may say
that the psycho-physical dispositions underlying the

great organic needs, nutrition (self-preservation) and reproduction, make use of a great variety of instincts in their service. Many of the instincts described by Dr. McDougall come into action in the pursuit of both self-preservative and race-preservative ends ; and it may be held that the reduction of the springs of conduct to fourteen primary instincts is not the ultimate analysis, or the only possible analysis, of the innate structure of the mind. The ends or goals pursued by the instincts are often only proximate ends, and are subordinate to the ultimate end of satisfying one of the great organic needs. But it is confusing to apply the term instinct to these organic needs if we continue to use the same term to indicate the innate dispositions to specific forms of behaviour, which alone constitute the instincts in Dr. McDougall's sense of the word.

Some of the misunderstanding and controversy about the importance ascribed to the sexual instinct in psycho-analytical writings may be traced to this source. On the one hand we have the loose use of the word instinct in everyday speech, and its more precise applications in psychology to instinctive behaviour in Dr. McDougall's sense, or, as in Mr. Shand's writings, to innately co-ordinated motor mechanisms ; on the other hand, we have Freud's extension of the term to everything innate in human nature that subserves in any way the final fulfilment or satisfaction of the needs of living organisms to reproduce themselves or to maintain and defend their individual existence. Moreover, in speaking of the sexual instinct, Freud does not confine himself to adult manifestations of the impulse whose final goal is the reproductive act, that is to say to the pairing or mating instinct in McDougall's terminology, but he includes within the purview of the " sexual instincts " all those tendencies of infancy and childhood which have genetic continuity with the mating instinct, and also certain impulses of adult life, such as those leading to the protection and love of children, which tend to secure the attainment of the ultimate goal of the mating instinct, namely, the survival and well-being of offspring, the continuance of the species, the preservation of the race.

But let us examine in more detail what Freud has in mind when he speaks of an instinct ; for he, like other writers on this topic, has a right to formulate his own notions of what an instinct may be, and his readers must for the time being accept his definitions or descriptions, however much they may disagree with them ; for only by bearing in mind what a writer means by any particular term can one get a true understanding of his point of view.

Freud approaches the problem of instinct from the physiological side, and he starts with the concept of stimulus and the scheme of the reflex arc. A stimulus from the outer world affecting living tissue is discharged by action towards the outer world. He conceives of an instinct as a stimulus to the mind, although not all mental stimuli are instinctual. Mental stimuli may come from the outside world, but they may also come from within the organism, and it is apparently only these latter that he regards as being of truly instinctual origin. Such stimuli cannot be avoided by flight or withdrawal as can those that come from without. An instinctual stimulus is a *need* which can be satisfied only by some inner change which takes away the need. ˎIndeed, it would seem as if Freud regards as instinctual only those innate dispositions which are stirred into activity by stimuli whose source is within the organism ; as if all that he would call instinct belonged to that class of instincts which Dr. Drever calls appetitive ; and he often seems to neglect or minimize the stimulus to instinctual activity that may come from the perception of an object. He says that an external stimulus acts as a single impact which calls out a single appropriate action, such as withdrawal from the source of stimulation ; an instinctual stimulus, on the other hand, always acts as a constant force from within, against which motor activity is of no avail.

Starting from this conception of an instinct, he speaks of its impetus, its aim, its object, and its source. The impetus is the motor element, the force of the impulse to activity inherent in every instinct-disposition. The aim of an instinct is satisfaction, brought about by getting rid of the condition which has given rise to the stimulus. In his recent works, however, Freud has had a good deal to say about instincts that are inhibited in respect of their aim. When this occurs it appears as if the instinct were allowed to go a certain length towards satisfaction, and is then inhibited so that its aim becomes deflected. The most important example of this is the change in the attitude of a child towards its parents which accompanies the repression of the Oedipus complex. The infantile sexual aims are renounced, yet the child remains tied to his parents by instincts which are the same as before, but are now inhibited in their aim. This is Freud's explanation of the origin of tender emotion, and he regards this inhibition of sexual aim as a form of sublimation and the most important element in love as contrasted with merely sensual desire.

The object of an instinct is that through which it can achieve its aim. The connexion between an instinct and its object is not very close, except where fixation has occurred. When there is no fixation the object of an instinct may be changed many times in the course of life. By the source of an instinct Freud means the bodily process, either physical or chemical, which provides the stimulus. It is therefore outside the province of psychology. On the question of classification of the instincts and the number that may be distinguished, Freud is not at all dogmatic. He says : " No objection can be made to anyone's employing the concept of an instinct of play or of destruction, or that of a social instinct, when the subject demands it and the limitations of psychological analysis allow of it. Nevertheless, we should not neglect to ask whether such instinctual motives, which are in one direction so highly specialized, do not admit of further analysis in respect of their sources, so that only those primal instincts which are not to be resolved further could really lay claim to the name." [1]

Considerations of this kind have led Freud to refuse to regard the herd-instinct as a primal instinct on the same level as the self-preservative and sexual instincts. Most writers who adopt a biological classification of the instincts accept the tri-partite division of them into self-preservative, race-preservative, and herd-instincts ; but Freud maintains that the herd-instinct is a derivative of the group of tendencies which he includes under the sexual instinct, being merely a development of the relationships which arise within the family.

During the greater part of the time when he was developing his psycho-analytic theory, Freud was content to accept the division of instincts into self-preservative and race-preservative, or Ego- and sexual

---

[1] Freud, *Collected Papers*, vol. iv, pp. 66–7.

instincts. It was a classification peculiarly congruent with the results of his analytic researches and supported by biological considerations of considerable weight. But when the conception of narcissistic Libido came to be entertained the antithesis of Ego-instincts and sexual instincts lost some of its force. Since narcissistic Libido is an expression of the energy of sexual instincts in the analytical sense, Freud says the sexual instincts must be "identified with the instincts of self-preservation". Part, at least, of the Ego-instincts is now recognized to be libidinal, and the contrast between Ego-instincts and sexual instincts is changed to one between *Ego*-instincts and *object*-instincts, both of which are of libidinal origin.

At this point our understanding of the position is rendered difficult by the fact that we have not yet come to any conclusion regarding the nature of Ego-instincts. Libido, we are told, becomes narcissistic when it is withdrawn from objects and turned towards the Ego. But it is not at all clear why any Ego-instincts should become libidinal merely because the Ego becomes an *object* of the Libido. If any Ego-instincts are libidinal we must suppose that they are so from the beginning, and not secondarily as a result of the narcissism which arises when the Libido of the Id withdraws from objects and turns towards the Ego.

But, however this may be, Freud does not consider all Ego-instincts to be libidinal, and he still maintains the contrast between libidinal and non-libidinal instincts. Libidinal instincts include object-instincts and some Ego-instincts ; the non-libidinal instincts consist of other instincts of the Ego.

The reasoning which led Freud to his latest views on the nature of the instincts is of a highly speculative character. It was forced upon him by his recognition of certain features of mental life which do not readily fit into the psycho-analytic doctrine that all mental functioning is automatically regulated by the pleasure-principle.

It was one of the earliest tenets of psycho-analysis that dream-formation is an outcome of the pleasure-principle, and that dreams, when interpreted, reveal themselves as disguised fulfilments of unconscious wishes. But during the war a class of dreams, known as battle-dreams, was met with in cases of so-called " shell-shock ", and these dreams when interpreted showed no evidence of wish-fulfilment ; they merely repeated the terrifying experience which had led to " nervous breakdown ". A similar tendency to repeat experiences that are not in themselves pleasurable may be observed in the play of children and in the life-histories of many apparently normal people. But perhaps the best example of this tendency to repetition is seen in the transference-situation which arises between patient and analyst in the course of treatment. Instead of recollecting various painful experiences of childhood the patient repeats them as current experiences in relation to the analyst. Frustration of instinctual impulses and desires, disappointments, jealousies, and failures in the sphere of the affections were the lot of childhood, but, notwithstanding the pain which accompanied them, these experiences are repeated in the transference with the same unpleasant consequences. Such repetition cannot be the work of the pleasure-principle, for some of these experiences could not at any time have been pleasurable. To account for such repetition of painful experiences Freud postulates, "beyond the pleasure-principle," a repetition-compulsion, "more primitive, more elementary, more instinctive than the pleasure-principle which is displaced by it."

From an examination of the part played by the repetition-compulsion in the traumatic neuroses Freud finds it to possess in a high degree an instinctual character. He finds in it something peculiar to all instincts—perhaps to all organic life—something in terms of which instinct may be defined, or, at least, described. In this connexion he defines instinct as "*a tendency innate in living organic matter impelling it towards the reinstatement of an earlier condition*".[1]

Freud takes a mechanistic view of the origin and nature of life and sees in the animation of inanimate matter merely the setting up of a tension which

---

[1] Freud, *Beyond the Pleasure Principle*, p. 44.

immediately strives to attain an equilibrium. Thus the
first instinct of life is a striving to return to lifeless-
ness—a death-instinct. And for primordial organisms
death would be easy and life would be short, until
external circumstances—the evolution of the earth
and its relation to the sun—forced upon them ever-
increasing deviations from the original path of life.
Seeing nothing in life itself but a disturbing tension
arising in the inanimate, Freud ascribes all increase of
structural and functional complexity in organisms to
these external forces ; and to the changes thus arising,
which he looks upon as but impediments to the return
to the inanimate, he ascribes all the phenomena of life
as we now know it. The course of life is but a circuitous
path to death, forced upon the organism in the
beginning by external forces and conserved for
repetition by the instincts.

According to this view the self-preservative
instincts—the Ego-instincts—are instincts which try
to secure that death shall come only in the way laid
down in the previous life-history of the race—" to secure
the path to death peculiar to the organism and to ward
off possibilities of return to the inorganic other than
the immanent ones." [1] A moment's consideration will
remind us that this cannot be the whole truth about
instinct. We may recall the teaching of Weismann,
that whilst all multicellular organisms die, the protista

[1] Freud, *Beyond the Pleasure Principle*, p. 48.

and the germ-plasm of higher organisms are potentially immortal.   Moreover, the facts of reproduction are a direct refutation of the view that the only goal of life is death.   When germ-cell and sperm-cell meet, a new repetition of an old cycle begins, which looks like a striving, not towards death, but towards life.   There must, therefore, be something in the nature of living organisms that is opposed to the death-instincts, for through the reproductive cells life is continuous from generation to generation.

But this continuance of life is only possible when union of male and female reproductive cells has taken place, and the strength of the life-impulse to achieve this end is manifested as the driving force behind all sexual activities.   The sexual instincts may, therefore, be regarded as life-instincts opposed to the death-instincts, as formerly they were opposed to the self-preservative or Ego-instincts.

In so far as the inanimate was in existence before the animate, the conception of death-instincts conforms to Freud's definition of instinct as a tendency towards the reinstatement of an earlier condition ; but it is not true of the individual organism to say that death is a reinstatement of an earlier condition unless we refer back the earlier condition to the very beginnings of life upon earth, or to the dust and ashes which by assimilation have become incorporate in the bodily organism of the individual.

The difficulty of making the definition apply to the life-instincts is still greater. For the aim of the life-instincts is the union of two cells and it does not seem possible that this can be a reinstatement of an earlier situation. At most it can only be a repetition of a chance conjugation of two protozoa. After examining various possibilities Freud confesses that science fails to provide any answer to the question : " Of what important happening in the process of development of the living substance is sexual repro-duction, or its forerunner, the copulation of two individual protozoa, the repetition ? " In quite another quarter, however, he finds a suggestion which, if it were in any sense true, would fulfil the conditions and would justify the statement that the life-instincts as well as the death-instincts are tendencies towards the reinstatement of earlier conditions. This suggestion he gets from the Myth of Aristophanes in Plato's *Symposium*—the myth of the round men whom Zeus cut in two. Just as in the myth the longing of lovers was explained as the longing of each for his own other half, so Freud would assume " that living substance was at the time of its animation rent into small particles which since that time strive for reunion by means of the sexual instincts ".

On this view every separate particle of living matter is endowed with Libido, with the life-instinct. Being living matter, however, it must also be subject to the death-instinct, the striving to get back to the inanimate. But the Libido pertaining to each individual cell of the body takes the other cells as its object, and by so doing it partially neutralizes the death-instincts of those cells and thus helps to keep them alive. In this way, Freud says, the Libido of our sexual instincts would coincide with the Eros of poets and philosophers, which holds together all living things.

Although it may be difficult to put forward the life-instincts as examples of the reinstatement of earlier conditions, it is at least easy to admit that the sexual instincts can appropriately enough be termed life-instincts. But we encounter a fresh difficulty when we try to find in actual operation any innate tendency which can properly be called a death-instinct ; for a death-instinct should tend towards the death of the organism, and no such tendency can be demonstrated. Here it might be said that, according to Freud's own reasoning, the death-instinct is manifested in the actual continuance of life ; for the instincts of self-preservation are merely "part-instincts designed to secure the path to death peculiar to the organism "— " even these watchmen of life were originally the myrmidons of death." But Freud himself does not put forward this defence, and when challenged to point to an example of a death-instinct his answer takes quite another form. He places alongside of the antithesis : life-instincts—death-instincts, another pair of opposites : love—hate, and he endeavours to bring these two polarities into relation with each other. He reminds us that a sadistic component of the sexual instinct has long been recognized ; " but how," he asks, " is one to derive the sadistic impulse, which aims at the injury of the object, from the life-sustaining Eros ?   Does not the assumption suggest itself that this sadism is properly a death-instinct, which is driven apart from the Ego by the influence of the narcissistic Libido, so that it becomes manifest only in reference to the object ? " [1]

Freud supposes that through the uniting of elementary unicellular organisms into multicellular forms of life, the death-instinct of the single cells has been neutralized and the impulses of destruction have been directed towards the outer world through the agency of the muscular system.   The death-instinct would thus manifest itself, in part at least, as an instinct of destruction in relation to the outer world and other forms of life.

In the beginning both life-instincts and death-instincts would be active, though unequally blended, in every piece of living substance ; and in later developments also we find fusions of the two kinds of instinct and also more or less complete separations of them.   In the sadistic component of the sexual instinct we find the instinct of destruction entering into the service of Eros to

[1] Freud, *Beyond the Pleasure Principle*, p. 69.

serve a useful purpose. In sadism, as a perversion, there is a separating out of this instinct so that it manifests independently.

In assimilating life-instincts and death-instincts to the polarity of love and hate, another difficulty is encountered. Clinical observation teaches us that not only does hate accompany love with unexpected regularity, not only is it often the forerunner of love in human relations, but that also there are many situations in which hate seems to turn into love or love into hate. Sometimes this change may be only temporal succession, the coming to fruition at different times of erotic and hostile tendencies ; but in studying the neuroses we sometimes meet what looks like an actual conversion of the one feeling into the other. It is as if energy were withdrawn from one impulse and conducted to the opposite one ; but a direct conversion of hate into love would seem to be incompatible with the qualitative difference between the two kinds of impulse. Freud, therefore, postulates the existence in the mental life of a supply of neutral or indifferent energy which can ally itself to an erotic or to a destructive impulse, different as these are in quality, and thus raise the total strength of the impulse, whether it be of love or of hate. This indifferent energy, which is so easily displaced, is derived, he thinks, from the store of narcissistic Libido—Libido which

I

in the process of becoming narcissistic has become desexualized.

From this rapid survey of Freud's Theory of the Instincts, we see that he is concerned with more elemental tendencies of living creatures than those to which the term instinct is usually applied. He makes little or no reference to the efforts of other psychologists to describe and classify what they believe to be the irreducible innate tendencies underlying human and animal behaviour. All his conclusions are based upon his analytical experience and a weighty criticism of the limitations of his method is that which points to his neglect of comparative psychology in his endeavours to solve such a problem as that of the instincts. But the psycho-analytical approach is so uniquely his own prescriptive right, and leads to such a novel and suggestive point of view, that psychologists of every school should welcome and treat with respect any conclusions that he may put forward. That these conclusions should have changed so considerably in the course of thirty years or more may be regarded as indicating that at the beginning of his researches he was not, as is often suggested, biassed in favour of any particular conception of the nature of the forces at work in the human mind. But at the beginning of his work one great group of primitive forces came into prominence at every step. In every case he examined he found himself listening to experiences related to the sexual life of the patient : to manifestations of the sexual instinct in the ordinary, everyday acceptation of the words. Further investigation led on to experiences of childhood genetically related to these adult experiences, and the tendencies underlying these experiences of childhood were, for good reasons, grouped under the sexual instincts. The conception of Libido, as the energy behind all manifestations of the sexual instinct in this extended sense of the word was formulated, and a distinction was drawn and an opposition recognized between self-preservative or Ego-instincts and race-preservative, sexual or libidinal instincts. The introduction of the concept of narcissism and narcissistic Libido did away with the opposition between Ego-instincts and Libido, for now it was seen that some Ego-instincts, self-preservative instincts, are also libidinal. The contrast now was between Libido directed towards the Ego and Libido directed towards objects. But here a new opposition came into view—an opposition between libidinal instincts (both Ego and object) and *other* Ego-instincts of which only one, the instinct of destruction, has been detected. Libidinal instincts, the sexual instincts, were opposed, as life-instincts, to hypothetical death-instincts, and the instinct of destruction was regarded as a death-instinct turned against the outer world, after being expelled from the Ego by the Libido. An extension of the Libido-concept to the individual cells of the body, whereby we conceive of each cell as taking the others as the object of its Libido, transforms the sexual instinct into the Eros which holds together all living things, and impels the particles of matter, rent asunder at the time of their animation, to come together again.

Two primordial instincts thus set in motion the whole drama of life : Eros, the life-instinct, the urge towards union of the living particles rent asunder when the inanimate became animate ; and the death-instinct, the striving towards the peace and quiet which seem to mortal eyes to reside in the inanimate.

A reader of Freud who sets out, as we have done, to discover what is meant by Ego-instincts may reasonably complain of their elusive nature. At no time do we find out what these Ego-instincts are and we get very little indication of what they do. Neither by approaching them from the side of the Ego nor from the side of the instincts are we able to bring the two halves of the term together in a way that carries any clear notion to the mind. The original antithesis between Ego and Libido encouraged us to hope that we might somewhere light upon a definition of Ego-instincts that would satisfy us ; but when analysis of the Ego brought us to the conclusion that much of the Ego itself is libidinal this opposition failed to be of value, and we became doubtful where to look for the ground of the conflict originally described as a struggle between the Ego and the Libido. We are, indeed, told, concerning the source of the opposition to the Libido, that it comes from the Ego-ideal, but it is not made clear how the mandates of the Ego-ideal are related to the instincts, or how the Ego-ideal itself is related to the Libido. At one time we think we are on the way to recognize the Ego-instincts, the self-preservative instincts, as the death-instincts, but this hope is destroyed by the discovery that the Ego-instincts are, in part at least, libidinal or life-instincts. Then we are expectant that the other Ego-instincts—those that are not libidinal—may be sufficient to uphold the original antithesis of Ego-instincts and Libido. But here, again, we seem to be disappointed, for the only Ego-instinct of a non-libidinal kind that analysis has so far been able to discover is the instinct of destruction—a death-instinct which manifests as an instinct of destruction only when it is expelled from the Ego by the Ego-libido.

Freud's Theory of the Instincts, in its final form. seems to take away all meaning from his earlier use of the term Ego-*instincts* to indicate the forces opposed to the Libido in the conflict giving rise to neurosis. It has always seemed an unhappy term, even when its meaning was only vaguely apprehended ; and now that analysis of the Ego has discriminated a differentiation within the Ego—the Ego-ideal or super-Ego—which is seen to be the actual source of the repressions, it should be unnecessary in the future to invoke Ego-*instincts* in explanation of endopsychic conflict.

THEORY OF THE NEUROSES

A LMOST everything of importance contributed by medical psychology to general psychology has been acquired through the study of the neuroses. The need to understand and describe the peculiarities of thinking, feeling, and doing, met with in these abnormal states has led to new conceptions of mental functioning which have proved to be of considerable value in the investigation of the normal mind, although they were at first neglected by psychologists on the ground that they applied only to abnormal conditions. The most important of these conceptions are the theory of mental dissociation expounded by Janet, and the kinds of mental process which Freud has described in his theory of the neuroses. It is, indeed, in the endeavour to formulate some consistent theory of the neuroses that investigators of the abnormal have made their most important contributions to psychology.

The separation of the neuroses as a group of disorders distinct from other maladies was a very late achievement of medical science, so that until comparatively recently there was no separate theory of the neuroses. Yet these disorders have been known from the beginnings of medicine, and throughout the centuries some kind of notion of their nature has been held.

119

We may recognize at least three phases of opinion concerning the nature of neurotic maladies. The first phase persisted from the days of Hippocrates down to those of Sydenham ; the next phase lasted from Sydenham to Charcot ; and the third phase, from Charcot to Freud, is that of our own time. The middle phase has left us nothing that is of much interest to us nowadays ; but, curiously enough, the dogma of the earlier period is found to have contained the essence of what many of us to-day believe to be the truth. What we may call the " theory of the neuroses " recorded by Plato in the *Timæus*, accepted literally by physicians for many centuries, and scoffed at in the age of enlightenment, comes to the front again in the teaching of Freud.

Plato, like Freud, had a theory of the Libido. " Wherefore also," he says, " in men the organ of generation becoming rebellious and masterful, like an animal disobedient to reason, seeks, by the raging of the appetites, to gain absolute sway ; and the same is the case with the so-called womb or matrix of women ; the animal within them is desirous of procreating children, and remaining unfruitful long beyond its proper time, gets discontented and angry, and, wandering in every direction through the body, closes up the passages of the breath, and, by obstructing respiration, drives them to extremity, causing all varieties of disease . . ." [1]

[1] *The Dialogues of Plato* (Jowett's trans.), vol. iii, p. 675.

That hysteria was considered to be in some way related to the sexual life is indicated by the name given to this malady, and although with the development of knowledge of anatomy any literal acceptation of Plato's words became impossible, and his theory consequently was pronounced absurd, nevertheless, the age-long belief in the connexion between neurotic ailments and disharmonies or dissatisfactions in the sexual life never really disappeared from medical tradition. Every acute observer—and there were many among the old-time practitioners of medicine—was aware of this connexion. But it was not taught in the schools, and young physicians and surgeons were in danger of losing touch with the wisdom of the ages in this matter. There was always a chance, however, that when they went out into the world and came in contact with older men they might hear something of this traditional knowledge. And this very often did happen. It happened to Freud, and he has recorded his astonishment on hearing, in private, from Charcot and other teachers, what they had never ventured to tell their students in the lecture room. Very early in my own medical career I had a similar experience, and on many occasions since then I have found this traditional knowledge of the connexion between neurosis and sexuality to be a common possession of the medical profession. Yet we know what an outcry was raised when Freud had the courage to proclaim this secret knowledge and to base it upon a scientific foundation ; and from none was the outcry louder than from the members of his own profession. Even to-day Freud's doctrines raise an amount of emotional heat in some people which is, I think, quite inexplicable unless these very doctrines themselves are invoked in explanation.

Before going on to consider Freud's theory of the neuroses, it is necessary to say a few more words about the views of Janet ; for Janet's writings form almost the only consistent scheme of psycho-pathology at the present time which is unaffected by Freud's teaching. Some reference will be made, in a subsequent lecture, to the theories of the neuroses put forward by writers like Jung and Adler, who have seceded from the school of Freud, and by those who, like Rivers and McDougall, have adopted some of Freud's views, but have not accepted the Libido-theory of the neuroses.

We have already, in our first lecture, considered the essential features of Janet's theory of the neuroses. He ascribes the occurrence of any and every form of psycho-neurotic illness to two main factors : (1) failure of the psychical tension which ordinarily acts as a synthesizing force and preserves the integrity of the " personal consciousness ", and (2) the liability of the tendencies most recently acquired, and of the acts most difficult of accomplishment, to become enfeebled or to drop away from the personal synthesis

when the psychical tension falls too low.   The
" tendencies " are, for Janet, of the nature of
mechanical reflexes, innate or acquired, and they do
not seem to carry any of the conative force or to have
the purposive nature which we ascribe to the instincts.
In his later writings, it is true, Janet's psychology has,
on the whole, become less subjective and mechanistic,
and more objective and dynamic, but the dynamism
is still a mechanical dynamism and not far removed
from behaviourism.

The diminution of psychical tension which leads to
neurosis is a result of exhaustion produced by emotion
or by excessive expenditure of energy in the accomplishment of acts belonging to a high order in the
hierarchy of the tendencies.   Janet does not admit
the part played by repression in inhibiting the output
of energy, and he seems to imply that all failure
to energize a particular act is always due to real
exhaustion.

Janet divides the neuroses into two great groups,
Hysteria and Psychasthenia.   As we have already seen,
he ascribes the symptoms of psychasthenia to a general
lowering of psychical tension whereby the highest and
most complicated mental functions are deprived of the
force necessary for their fulfilment.   In hysteria, for
reasons which he has insufficiently explained, the
lowering of the level of psychical tension is localized,
so that, instead of a general diminution of function,

there is a retraction of the field of consciousness and a consequent mental dissociation.

Perhaps the most important and most permanent part of Janet's work in abnormal psychology is his wonderful series of studies on the dissociations of hysteria ; more especially of those massive dissociations which become manifest as somnambulisms, fugues, and multiple personalities. In this same department of abnormal psychology, and worthy of being ranked alongside of Janet's studies, we place the works of Dr. Morton Prince ; and the contributions of both these writers to the psychology of dissociation provide certain problems which up to the present have been inadequately dealt with by the psycho-analysts. Moreover, it is just on this topic of dissociation that the initial divergence of the theories of Freud from those of Janet is to be found. For Janet, dissociation is a merely mechanical splitting of the mind due to lack of the psychical tension which ordinarily keeps it together. For Freud, dissociation is a rending of the mind by dynamic forces within itself.

The most fundamental concept of Freudian psychology is that of mental conflict and repression. Everything else is secondary and derivative. The notion of conflict within the mind is in itself not peculiar to psycho-analytical psychology. We meet with it in Herbart as a conflict between *ideas* for the privilege of entering consciousness. But Freud has made the conflict a real conflict between incompatible motives or between impulses towards incompatible goals. whereas the "ideas" of Herbart's intellectualistic system possess no driving power which can lead to struggle of any kind.

We have already spoken of the kinds of impulses which Freud found to be engaged in the conflicts and repressions that lead to neurosis ; and we have examined in outline the various mental processes which take place between the original act of repression and the formation of neurotic symptoms. We have seen that the starting point of neurotic disturbances may be found in some form of privation of libidinal satisfaction, although whether privation does or does not lead to neurosis in any individual depends upon other factors. The chief of these factors is the presence or absence of those fixations which the Libido may suffer in the course of its development.

As in physical illness we speak of exciting causes and predisposing causes, so in the neuroses we may say that privation is the exciting cause and fixation is the predisposing cause. The predisposition resulting from Libido-fixation may be regarded as a constitutional factor, although it is a factor which is partly inherited and partly acquired in childhood. The part that is acquired in childhood may be regarded as truly constitutional in the adult, for, before neurosis sets in, it has become part of the structure of the mind and helps to determine the way in which the organism as a whole reacts to the stress of privation.

The hereditary predisposition to neurosis would seem to be entirely a matter of the innate sexual constitution ; the acquired predisposition depends upon accidental experiences in childhood which lead to fixation and thus disturb the normal course of Libido-development. The exciting causes of neurosis are events or circumstances in adult life which help to bring about privation of libidinal satisfaction and a consequent introversion and regression of Libido. But, besides the hereditary or acquired constitutional factor and the external factor of privation, there is a third factor— susceptibility to conflict—on which the outbreak of neurosis ultimately depends.

Let us recall, once more, the course of events which Freud's theory of the neuroses implies. First of all there is privation resulting in accumulation of Libido which cannot be disposed of by sublimation or by any other form of substitution. The pent-up Libido, turning away from possibilities of satisfaction in the outer world, becomes introverted and reanimates phantasies which until now may have been tolerated because they were so lightly charged with Libido that there was no danger of their being transformed into actualities. The phantasies thus reanimated by the introverted Libido press towards realization and come into conflict with the Ego. And here, just depending on the kind of development which has taken place in the Ego, we meet with variations in the third factor necessary for the outbreak of neurosis—the susceptibility to conflict.

The development of the Ego, like the development of the Libido, may become arrested, and that differentiation within the Ego, which Freud has called the super-Ego or Ego-ideal, may be slight or non-existent. If the Ego remains at the childhood stage and does not repudiate infantile forms of sexual gratification or infantile love-objects, the phantasies may be allowed to become actualities and gratification in some form of perversion may be obtained. But when an Ego-ideal has arisen, when there is within the Ego some ideal of conduct which renders abhorent the kinds of gratification suggested by the phantasies, then the phantasies are repressed and the Libido finds its way back to the fixation-points from which the phantasies originally arose. The ungratified Libido would thus seem to be farther off than ever from achieving satisfaction ; but it is now wholly unconscious, and it can take advantage of the special processes characteristic of the unconscious system of the mind by means of which neurotic symptoms are produced. By way of displacement and condensation the now unconscious wish-phantasy can attain a surrogate satisfaction in the symptom. But the Ego takes care that its own wishes also are represented, and the symptom stands for denial and self-punishment as well as for gratification.

Sometimes the gratification, sometimes the denial, is the more prominent element in the symptom, and the accent falls on the one rather than on the other, according to the kind of neurosis which develops. Freud says :   " The purpose of the symptom is either a sexual gratification or a defence against it ; in hysteria the positive, wish-fulfilling character predominates on the whole, and in the obsessional neurosis the negative ascetic character . . . In hysteria a collaboration of the two tendencies in one symptom is usually achieved. In the obsessional neurosis the two parts are often distinct ; the symptom is then a double one, and consists of two successive actions which cancel each other." [1]

The points of fixation to which the Libido regresses seem to stamp the symptoms with the characteristics that lead us to classify the neuroses and to divide them into groups or types to which distinctive names are given. The chief of these have already been referred to. We may recall also that regression may take the form of a return to early love-objects or a return to infantile modes of gratification, that is to say, to gratification appropriate to an earlier stage of Libido-organization. The latter form of regression is characteristic of obsessional neurosis and determines the kind of symptoms met with in this disorder. Fixation has taken place at the sadistic-anal stage of Libido-development, and the love-impulses which enter into the obsessional thoughts take the form of a desire to kill the loved

[1] Freud, *Introductory Lectures*, p. 253.

person.   The infantile sadism dominates the unconscious love-attitude and it emerges in consciousness as an obsessional or compulsive thought.   The horror occasioned by such an obsession may be intensified by the fact that regression to early love-objects may also have occurred, so that the impulse to kill is directed against the parents, or brothers, or sisters.

But regression to early love-objects is more noticeable in hysteria, for here the picture is not blurred by return to the pre-genital stage of Libido-organization.   In hysteria the genital stage of development has been reached, and even though the dawning of adult sexuality has been repressed so that, as often happens, the sexual instinct of the hysteric may be described as lacking, nevertheless it exists in the unconscious in its adult form.   And when the Libido regresses to the Oedipus fixation, the unconscious relation to the love-object is a truly incestuous one, for it takes the form imposed upon it by the adult genital organization.   One consequence of this is that repression plays the principal part in the production of hysteria, whereas in the production of obsessional neurosis regression to the pre-genital stage is the chief factor.

In dementia praecox and other psychoses the fixation-points to which the Libido regresses are farther back in the developmental history of the Libido than those of hysteria and obsessional neurosis.   The weak spot is probably at the stage of primary narcissism.

The phantasies which prove to be pathogenic and which are represented in the symptoms are built upon the desires and impulses related to the stage of Libido-development at which fixation has taken place.   In the course of analysis, in the interpretation of the meaning of the symptoms, these phantasies come to light. They may be told as actual experiences of childhood or infancy, and it is often impossible to decide whether they have been actual experiences or are merely the products of phantasy.   Freud, in his early work, took them at their face value, and believed that his patients had actually had the infantile experiences which they related to him in analysis. Later, however, he became convinced that as a rule these scenes of infancy were not real experiences, and that sometimes they were in direct opposition to what the actual experiences had been.   Yet sometimes the episodes described had been actual occurrences, although in other cases exactly similar descriptions proved to be nothing but phantasies.

For example, stories of seduction in childhood occurred very frequently in Freud's early analyses, and he tells us that he over-estimated the frequency of such occurrences because he had not yet learnt to discriminate between phantasies and the memories of actual happenings. On the other hand, seduction of children does often actually occur and may form the starting point of a neurosis.   Further experience of neurotic patients did not lessen the frequency of such stories, and it came to be realized that, although they very often were phantasies and not memories of actual experiences, they nevertheless played the same important part in the production of neurosis as had been originally ascribed to them.[1]

It is now recognized that certain phantasies of infantile experience, such as seduction, castration, and the witnessing of parental intercourse, recur again and again in the analysis of neurotic disorders ; and Freud has come to the conclusion that " childhood experiences of this kind are in some way necessarily required by the neurosis . . . If they can be found in real events, well and good ; but if reality has not supplied them they will be evolved out of hints and elaborated by phantasy ".[2]

Thus it happens that we meet with the same phantasies again and again, in the analysis of different patients. And just as there are these typical phantasies, so there are certain symptoms which may be called typical. Such symptoms as the phobias of anxiety-hysteria are fundamentally very much alike in every case, although in each patient there is some difference which depends on circumstances and experiences in his personal life.   These individual

[1] Melanie Klein's work shows that most of these probably *were* real experiences (between children), but falsely ascribed by wish-fulfilment to the adult environment.

[2] Freud, *Introductory Lectures*, p. 310.

features can be interpreted in the light of repressed
material related to the personal history, whereas the
typical elements in the symptoms are resistent to such
historical interpretation.   A similar difficulty is
encountered in the interpretation of dreams. Many of
the symbols employed in the making of dreams seem
to have some universal significance and occur in the
dreams of everyone ; and here, also, we find that such
dreams cannot be interpreted from the associations
supplied by the dreamer, but can be understood only
in the light of knowledge of the meaning of symbols
which has been obtained from other sources.

   In explanation of all these peculiarities of the mental
life—typical dreams and dream-symbols, typical
symptoms, typical phantasies—Freud is inclined to
adopt a view which is thought by many to be open to
grave objections. He thinks that just as the individual
features of dream, of symptom-formation, and of
phantasy are derived from and can be explained by
personal experiences, so the typical features, common
to large numbers of people, are derived from the
experience of the race and can be explained only as
a racial inheritance.   He thinks, for example, that
certain phantasies such as those of seduction and
castration—the primal phantasies as he calls them—
are a phylogenetic possession ; that " all that to-day
is narrated in analysis in the form of phantasy . . was
in prehistoric periods of the human family a reality " ;

and that " the child in its phantasy simply fills out the gaps in its true individual experiences with true pre-historic experiences ". He is of opinion " that more knowledge of the primordial forms of human development is stored up for us in the psychology of the neuroses than in any other field we may explore ".[1] Freud does not go into any detail on this question of hereditary transmission of mental dispositions, but there is throughout all his work an obvious leaning towards Lamarckian doctrines.   If experience, or the psycho-physical dispositions laid down by experience, are not transmissible, he does not see how there could ever have been any progress.   Yet he admits that the experiences of the Ego seem to be lost as far as heredity is concerned, but he thinks that if they are repeated often and strongly enough in many individuals through successive generations, they are converted into experiences of the Id ; and that the impressions thus made upon the Id are transmitted as innate mental dispositions.

Everything known about the causes giving rise to neurosis points to the truth of Freud's formula : Neurosis is the result of a conflict between the Ego and its Id. His later researches have led him to a contrasting formula about the causation of psychosis : psychosis is the result of a conflict between the Ego and its environment (the outer world). In neurosis the Ego repudiates and represses the powerful instinctual

[1] Freud, *Introductory Lectures*, p. 310.

impulses derived from the Id which are pressing for gratification by converting the phantasies into actual experiences. The Ego initiates the repression at the instigation of the Ego-ideal, and the dictates of the Ego-ideal prove stronger than the instinctual demands of the Id. The repressed impulses struggle against the Ego, and, through the mechanisms of condensation and displacement, succeed in obtaining a surrogate satisfaction in the symptoms. The Ego then continues the struggle against the symptoms. In psychosis, on the other hand, the Ego, in conflict with its environment, submits to the domination of the Id and is perforce compelled to sever its relation to the outer world and repudiate the claims of reality. Interest in the outer world is lost, and a new world, a new reality, is created by the Ego by means of hallucination and delusion.

In neurosis there is frustration by the claims of reality, represented by the outer world or the Ego-ideal, and the Ego takes sides with reality and repudiates the Id. In psychosis there is frustration also, but here the Ego is overwhelmed by the Id, and is torn away or withdraws itself from reality. Bearing in mind, however, the threefold relation of the Ego to its ideal, its Id, and its outer world, we see that there is another possible field of conflict, namely a conflict between the Ego and its Ego-ideal. Freud thinks that the results of analysis justify us in recognizing conditions arising from such a conflict, and he places melancholia in this group, which he would like to call the narcissistic psycho-neuroses ; for the most salient feature of melancholia is the self-condemnation resulting from the severity of the Ego-ideal towards the Ego.

Thus, Freud says, " a transference neurosis corresponds to a conflict between Ego and Id, a narcissistic neurosis to that between Ego and super-Ego, and a psychosis to that between Ego and outer world." [1]

These are recent formulations in psycho-analytic theory and they are put forward by Freud tentatively as hypotheses which may be more fully verified by further investigation. He has often, in the course of the development of his theory of the neuroses, had occasion to modify or correct his earlier conclusions, and this is indeed one of his great merits ; but it is one of the reasons why it is difficult to get a clear grasp of his recent teaching and to reconcile his present views with what he taught in earlier days. A noticeable instance of this is to be found in his latest views on the source of the morbid anxiety which is so commonly suffered by all neurotic patients.

We have seen that the symptoms of all the transference neuroses appear to be means of protecting the Ego from anxiety. It looks, we said, as if the Ego were afraid of the Libido. But morbid anxiety is not conspicuous until after repression has occurred ; therefore, it was thought that the immediate fate of repressed

[1] Freud, *Collected Papers*, vol. ii, p. 254.

Libido is its conversion into anxiety, or, rather, its discharge in the form of anxiety. In the formation of a neurosis various processes occur which tend to prevent the development of such anxiety. In the phobias, for example, the anxiety supposed to come from the repressed Libido is projected on some external object, and precautions and safeguards are then adopted by which the dangerous object may be avoided.

Freud has now given up this explanation of the origin of morbid anxiety; he no longer teaches that repressed Libido becomes converted into anxiety or secures discharge in this way. He seems to have returned to the more intelligible view that morbid anxiety, like real anxiety, is an affective reaction of the Ego to danger. The difference is that real anxiety is a reaction to real danger, danger that we are conscious of; whereas morbid anxiety arises from a danger which we do not consciously recognize, a danger from the unconsciously anticipated consequences of gratifying instinctual impulses. Thus, morbid anxiety is not a consequence of repression; on the contrary, repression may be the first response of the Ego to the danger signal.[1]

The prototype of danger to the Ego is found in the experience of birth, the experience of utter helpless-

---

[1] Dr. Ernest Jones has all along taught that morbid anxiety is derived from the Ego as a defensive reaction to repressed Libido. See his *Collected Papers on Psychoanalyis*.

ness on being separated from the mother. This causes the first anxiety-reaction, a reaction which in the circumstances is adequate ; for the infant's yelling is a means of preventing the poisoning of the blood which threatens when separation from the mother at birth occurs. The infant at birth suffers its first privation, some of its needs are being frustrated and it reacts with anxiety.

A similar situation—separation from the mother— is repeated on many occasions throughout the child's life. The earliest fears of childhood, the fear of being alone, the fear of being in the dark, the fear of being with strangers, all refer to the absence of the loved mother. But here, as in the privation caused by separation from the mother at birth, the danger threatened is the loss of gratification of some of the child's needs. Such privation leads to an increase of psychical tension, and this culminates in the anxiety-reaction of yelling for the mother. As the child grows older the absence of the mother causes the anxiety-reaction before increased tension actually occurs. Here anxiety is being used as a signal to ward off a danger which has not yet appeared.

This is comparable to the function of anxiety in the production of a neurosis. The Ego anticipates danger from loss of a love-object, or from punishment (e.g. castration) for libidinal wishes, or from anger and loss of love from the super-Ego. It therefore sets up defences to guard itself from these dangers, and these defences sometimes issue in the establishment of a neurosis.

The concept of defence was one of the earliest achievements of psycho-analytic theory ; but, since in hysteria the defence is so invariably carried out by means of repression, and since the first cases to be investigated were all cases of this disorder, the more general concept of defence was largely given up and was replaced by the more specific one of repression. But it is now recognized that repression is but one of the ways in which defence may be accomplished. In obsessional neurosis the regression of the libido and the reaction-formations are in themselves mechanisms of defence, as are also certain Ego-activities, peculiar to this neurosis, which play a part in the formation of the symptoms.

Let me summarize as briefly as possible the Libido-theory of the neurosis. The Libido is the energy of the sexual instincts at all ages in the life-history of the individual. It passes through various developmental phases in each of which it is related to different parts or organs of the body. It becomes organized successively in the organs of nutrition, excretion, and generation. Normally its organization passes on from one stage to another until it assumes its final adult form, but sometimes it lingers too long at one of the early stages, and is then said to suffer fixation. As a result of fixation the volume of Libido that goes on to adult organization is diminished, and consequently there is a lessening of the energy available for achieving Libido-satisfaction in later life. Thus frustration of adult Libido-satisfaction more readily occurs, and frustration, however brought about, results in privation.

Besides the development of organization in different parts or organs of the body, the Libido undergoes development in respect of the objects towards which it is directed and from which it obtains satisfaction. At the narcissistic stage the object of the Libido is the child's own body. At the stage of object-love proper the parents and, later, brothers and sisters, are the first objects of the Libido. If there is no Oedipus fixation the love-life develops normally and the Libido then finds its objects in the outer world, outside the family. But, if through force of circumstances, or inner inhibitions, or feebleness of the Libido due to fixation, a normal love-life is not achieved, then the Libido suffers frustration and privation ensues.

But by many people privation is not well borne, and the Libido that is frustrated by reality turns back in introversion to the phantasies. The roots of the phantasies are found in two directions—in activities related to earlier forms of Libido-organization and in the love-objects of infantile life ; and when introversion occurs the Libido may regress towards one or other or both of these roots.

While the Libido is passing through the various stages in its development there is a parallel development of the Ego. Arising originally in response to the claims of reality impressed upon the organism through the perceptual system, the Ego at first ministers to the needs of the Libido and tries to secure for them real satisfactions. But the claims of reality are soon found to be incompatible with gratifications of the Libido, and a differentiation within the Ego, an Ego-ideal, arises by identification with the parent whose opposition to Libido-strivings is the chief obstacle in the way of their satisfaction. The growth of the Ego-ideal and the severity of its attitude towards the Libido depends on the kind of environment into which the child is born—on the cultural atmosphere of the home, the æsthetic and moral standards of the parents, and the conventions imposed by the social requirements of the time and place. The degree of oppositon between the Ego-ideal and Libido-strivings is the measure of that susceptibility to mental conflict and repression which is the forerunner and the main determinant of neurosis.

When, in consequence of privation, the Libido becomes introverted and regresses to the phantasies, there is danger that the phantasies thus reanimated may be converted into actual experiences ; but any tendency in the Ego to allow such gratification of the Libido is met by such opposition as the Ego-ideal is fitted to afford. If a high ideal has been formed, the severity of the Ego-ideal will compel the Ego to repress the unworthy or reprehensible phantasies, and the Libido will then retreat to the fixation-points in the unconscious which are the roots from which the phantasies originally grew.

The repressed Libido, now entirely unconscious, takes advantage of the mental processes peculiar to the unconscious, and by means of condensation and displacement, and consequent distortion and disguise, can secure some sort of satisfaction in neurotic symptoms which are symbolic substitutes for repressed libidinal wishes. But even here the ban of the Ego-ideal is in evidence, for the symptom is at best but a compromise, and in the symptom the Ego is compelled to suffer a punishment inflicted by the Ego-ideal.

THE APPLICATIONS OF MEDICAL PSYCHOLOGY

THE knowledge acquired in the investigation of
the neuroses finds its most immediate application
in the treatment of these disorders. It was in pursuit
of this therapeutic aim that medical psychology
originated, and although there is hardly any branch of
mental or social science that has not been influenced by
its doctrines, it still finds its most important field of
practical usefulness in psycho-therapeutics. One of the
consequences of this is that the value of each new
discovery is apt to be judged by its usefulness in the
treatment of morbid states. But in medical psychology,
as in other departments of science, immediate utility
is not a good test of the importance of a discovery.
Practical utility may be the final test of the value of
any new piece of knowledge, but it cannot be accepted
as the immediate test ; if it were so, some of the greatest
discoveries of science would have been rejected at their
birth. So we cannot judge the importance of the
concepts of medical psychology by the success, or want
of success, which attends their therapeutic application.
We should judge rather by the range of their application
in other directions, such as, for example, the degree

in which they enable us to understand human behaviour, either normal or abnormal.

If it is a mistake to make immediate practical utility a test of the value of a discovery, it is a still greater mistake to make it a test of its truth. Nowhere is the pragmatic test of truth more liable to mislead than in the sphere of psycho-therapeutics. If you hold a certain view about the nature of hysterical symptoms, and take remedial measures in accordance with that view, the symptoms may disappear ; but this does not by any mean show that your view of the nature of hysteria is a true one. If it did so, then it might be said that every opinion that has ever been put forward in explanation of hysteria must be true, for hysterical symptoms have disappeared under every form of treatment that has ever been tried.

In dealing with the applications of medical psychology it is necessary to draw a dividing line between Freudian and pre-Freudian conceptions, or, as we may say, between the psycho-analytic and the hypnotic periods of investigation and treatment. The hypnotic period contributed little of importance to psychology apart from the theory of dissociation and the abundant evidence which it provided of the far-reaching influence of suggestion. From a practical point of view, the latter is the more important, but owing to imperfect theoretical understanding of the nature of suggestion, many false notions found currency about the part played by suggestion in ordinary life and about the structure and functioning of the normal mind.

It was observed that in a person who had been subjected to a course of hypnotic experiment there appeared to be a doubling of the stream of consciousness. Besides the normal waking consciousness, there seemed to be a hypnotic stratum which was sometimes referred to as the subconscious or subliminal. This was supposed to be the part of the mind which carried out hypnotic and post-hypnotic suggestions, and since it was found that all people, or nearly all people, are suggestible in some degree, it was assumed that everyone had a subconsciousness capable of functioning in the same way as the secondary consciousness revealed in hypnotic experiment. On this view the mind was regarded as comprising two separate streams of thought which flowed side by side, the chief difference between them being that the primary stream could be influenced by reason whereas the secondary stream was only open to suggestion.

The principal error in this view is the failure to recognize that when hypnosis is induced, and more especially when it is frequently induced, for the purposes of treatment or experiment, an artificial dissociation is brought about and a more or less fleeting secondary personality is formed ; so that during the period of hypnotic influence, that is to say, during the whole

L

of the time that the experiments are going on, the mind of the hypnotic subject is not in a normal state, however normal he may appear to be when attending to the affairs of everyday life. There is present in him a mental dissociation of a kind which we have no reason to believe exists in the minds of normal people.

Yet, although these phenomena of dissociation are not found in ordinary healthy people, the study of them has led to a much fuller understanding than was formerly possible of certain types of behaviour which, though not commonly regarded as abnormal, are nevertheless unusual and out of the ordinary. The trance states of mystics and visionaries, some of the seemingly supernormal phenomena of so-called mediums, automatic writing and other forms of motor automatism, crystal gazing, hallucinations and illusions in the sane, and many of the productions of literary and artistic genius, have all had much light thrown upon them by the psychology of mental dissociation.

The therapeutic practice of the pre-Freudian period was almost entirely confined to treatment by suggestion ; or to methods introduced as substitutes for suggestion, in which, nevertheless, suggestion played the chief part. Of these, perhaps the most interesting is what was called treatment by persuasion. Hypnotic practice was in its day opposed by the orthodox as violently as psycho-analytic practice has been in recent years. Hypnotism was declared to be an

" unclean thing ", and suggestion without hypnosis was felt to be too like the waving of a magician's wand to be respectable. Some physicians who took up this attitude towards hypnosis and suggestion nevertheless realized that neurotic disorders must be treated through the mind ; and, since they recognized that the behaviour of neurotics as revealed in their symptoms is " unreasonable ", they set themselves to appeal to the reason of their patients, to explain to them the nature of their disabilities, to convince them that they could, if they would, get free from them, and to coax or command them to do so.

By these means many neurotic sufferers were relieved, and the exponents of this method declared that their results were due to *persuasion* ; that is to say, to a successful appeal to the reason of the patient.

We know now that this is not the true explanation. A neurotic symptom is unconsciously determined and no appeal to the reason has any effect upon it. But in making an appeal to the reason, in seeking to convince and to persuade, we cannot avoid the subtle action of suggestion ; and suggestion, being a form of appeal to the unconscious, has, when successful, the same result in treatment by persuasion as it has in treatment by hypnotism.

By far the most important problem presented by all forms of treatment used in pre-analytical days is the nature and source of suggestion. But the theory of dissociation gave no very satisfying explanation. For Janet suggestion consists in the setting in action of a dissociated system. It produces its results by "artificially causing, in the form of impulsion, the functioning of a tendency that the subject cannot obtain in the form of a personal will". But the tendencies, for Janet, are merely tendencies towards a series of co-ordinated movements, innate or acquired by habit, and bear little relation to the instinctive conations which lead to purposive behaviour. He never gets quite free from the old notion of ideo-motor action. What gives the impulsion its force is the full development of the suggested idea, owing to its dissociation from the rest of the personality. Being isolated from all inhibiting ideas, it is unreflectingly assented to and takes the form of an impulse.

In this explanation Janet gives no place to what should be regarded as the main factors in suggestion, namely, the personal influence of the operator and the affective state of *rapport* in the subject. It is true he recognizes the existence of such personal influence and admits its importance in treatment, but he considers it (under the designation of "direction") as something distinct from suggestion and independent of it. He admits that there is a close relationship between the two, but he does not believe they are the same or that the one is inseparable from the other.

Freud's theory of suggestion differs fundamentally

from that of Janet in so far as he lays stress here, as elsewhere, on the purposive nature of all mental activity and on the importance of affective states. *Rapport* is the essence of hypnosis, and the factors giving rise to *rapport* come into play in all suggestion, whether in the hypnotic or the waking state. Quite early in his psycho-analytic experience Freud came to the conclusion that the nature of hypnosis is attributable to the unconscious fixation of the Libido on the person of the hypnotizer. Ferenczi elaborated this view, and maintained that the capacity to be hypnotized and influenced by suggestion depends on the possibility of transference taking place ; that is to say, on the displacement on to the hypnotist of the unconscious libidinal attitude towards the parents or parent-substitutes. Referring to the two ways of giving suggestion, he said that the hypnotist with imposing appearance who gives his suggestions in the form of commands recalls the stern, all-powerful, father, and that, in the other method of giving suggestion, the gentle monotonous words and the stroking hand are reminiscent of the tender mother. The hypnotist arouses in the hypnotized person the same feelings of love or fear and the same conviction of infallibility as had been aroused in him by his parents when he was a child. The feelings and desires still attached to the parents in the unconscious are transferred to the hypnotist, and provide the motive force for hypnotic credulity and compliance.   The hypnotized person is really unconsciously in love with the hypnotist.

Freud himself has, more recently, dealt fully with the Libido-theory of hypnosis and suggestion. In doing so he reminds us of the psycho-analytical use of the term *Libido*. He says : " We call by that name the energy . . . . of those instincts which have to do with all that may be comprised under the word ' love '. The nucleus of what we mean by love naturally consists . . . in sexual love with sexual union as its aim.   But we do not separate from this . . . on the one hand, self-love, and on the other, love for parents and children, friendship and love for humanity in general, and also devotion to concrete objects and to abstract ideas.   Our justification lies in the fact that . . . . all these tendencies are an expression of the same instinctive activities ; in relations between the sexes these instincts force their way towards sexual union, but in other circumstances they are diverted from their aim or are prevented from reaching it, though always preserving enough of their original nature to keep their identity recognizable (as in such features as the longing for proximity and self-sacrifice)." [1]   Instincts which are thus inhibited in their aim are accompanied by, or give rise to, emotions which have no longer a sensual character, but show varying degrees of love in the form of tenderness, devotion, or friendliness.

[1] Freud, *Group Psychology and the Analysis of the Ego*, pp. 37–8.

Freud says that in the state of being in love the narcissistic Libido ordinarily attached to the Ego-ideal is displaced on to the loved person whose merits are proportionately over-estimated. The lover projects part of his narcissism and thereby loses the self-confidence which narcissism sustains; he becomes humble and unassuming, while the loved person becomes idealized so as to appear free from imperfection and incapable of doing wrong. The criticizing function of the Ego-ideal is abrogated, and conscience does not enter into what is done for the sake of the beloved. As Freud says: "The whole situation can be completely summarized in a formula; the object has taken the place of the Ego-ideal"

It was just this over-estimation of the loved person, and the consequent acquiescence in his judgments and blind obedience to his wishes, that led Freud to explain the nature of hypnosis by the unconscious fixation of Libido on the person of the hypnotizer. The recognition of a Libido-relation between the hypnotized person and the hypnotist carried the implication that this is a love-relation of some kind, although this aspect was not emphasized by Freud at that time. Now, however, he says quite frankly: "From being in love to hypnosis is evidently only a short step. The respects in which the two agree are obvious. There is the same humble subjection, the same compliance, the same absence of criticism towards the hypnotist just as towards the

loved object . . . no one can doubt that the hypnotist
has stepped into the place of the Ego-ideal."

The main question at issue in considering the
psycho-analytic theory of suggestion and hypnosis
is whether the state of *rapport* is or is not a libidinal
manifestation. Various alternative theories have been
put forward.   Trotter, for example, derives all
suggestibility from a herd-instinct, gregariousness,
which he regards as a primitive and fundamental
quality in man. Gregariousness implies an extreme
sensitiveness of every individual to the behaviour of
the herd, and is, in Trotter's view, the basis of all
human suggestibility. Variations in susceptibility to
suggestion are explained as being due to the different
extent to which suggestions are identified with the
voice of the herd. If we were convinced that all
behaviour which Trotter ascribes to herd-instinct is
really due to a primary instinctual impulse of this
nature, we might agree with his view that suggestion
also is a manifestation of the herd-instinct.   How
powerful the driving force derived from such a source
would be is clearly seen in the emotional and compulsive nature of the acts performed under its
instigation. But there are good grounds for believing
that the gregarious instinct is not irreducible, as
Trotter maintains, but can be traced to its roots in the
child-parent relation and the group relations of the
family.   The dispositions to such relations within the

family are probably an archaic inheritance and are the bearers of tendencies appropriate to the prehistoric form of family life which probably consisted of a horde led by a horde-father.

The herd-instinct theory of suggestion finds little support from the phenomena of hypnotic suggestion. The influence of the herd would here seem to be more than ordinarily excluded, and the relation between the hypnotized person and the hypnotist appears to be of an intimately personal kind.

Another explanation of hypnotic credulity and obedience is given by Professor McDougall in the theory of suggestion which he put forward in his *Social Psychology* and still adheres to in his recently published *Outline of Abnormal Psychology*. From observation that among gregarious animals we find relations of dominance and submission, McDougall argues that the tendency of some members of a herd to submit tamely and quietly to the dominance of a leader is instinctive, and that such behaviour is the expression of a distinct and specific instinct of submission which is evoked by the aggressive or self-assertive behaviour of older and stronger members of the herd. Human beings also are endowed with this instinct and in them it is similarly evoked by those who give evidence of superiority or have a reputation for power. McDougall maintains that " the impulse, the emotional conative tendency of this instinct, is the

main conative factor at work in all instances of true
suggestion ; whether waking or hypnotic ". He dissents
from the view of Trotter that suggestion is sufficiently
accounted for by invoking the herd-instinct, for he
holds that gregarious and submissive tendencies are
independent variables and cannot be ascribed to the
same instinct.

In McDougall's theory of suggestion *rapport* between
the operator and the hypnotic subject is essentially the
relation of prestige and submission which renders
possible all waking suggestion ; but for the hypnotic
subject the prestige of the operator is indefinitely
increased by the success of the latter's suggestions ;
and the docility of the former is correspondingly
augmented.

The theories of both Trotter and McDougall agree
with the theory of Freud in so far as all three invoke
an impulse of submission as the main conative factor
in suggestion ; but McDougall regards submission as
a primary instinct, Trotter looks upon it as a derivative
of the gregarious instinct, and Freud ascribes it to what
he has called the masochistic component of the sexual
instinct. According to his recent speculations, however,
masochism is not itself of sexual origin ; it arises from
that part of the death-instinct which has not been
turned outwards in the form of sadism, but has become
bound up with, and entered into the service of, the
Libido which has tried to master it. *Rapport,* in

McDougall's opinion is a prestige-relation ; in that of Freud it is a love-relation.

Had we no way of deciding between these two views, we might be content to accept either of them as affording a reasonable explanation of the phenomena of *rapport* and suggestion. But we have a way of discovering the nature of the patient's affective attitude towards the hypnotist which manifests as *rapport* and is the basis of effective suggestion. Psycho-analysis gives us proof, in two ways, that this attitude is a love-attitude, a form of libidinal tie. In the first place some patients who have been treated by hypnotic suggestion have subsequently been analysed and the love-attitude in hypnotic *rapport* has been clearly shown. In the second place it is found that in the course of every analysis a similar relation between patient and analyst arises. The transference-relation in analysis begins in exactly the same way as the *rapport*-relation in hypnosis, namely, by an unconscious fixation of Libido on the person of the physician. The only difference is that in the hypnotic subject this direction of the Libido may remain throughout uncon-scious, whereas in analysis it is forced to become conscious and its origin in " transference " is laid bare ; that is to say, its origin in displacement of Libido from its attachment to the love-objects of the phantasies and its transference to the analyst.

I have dwelt on this topic of *rapport* or, as we shall

henceforth call it, transference because it is the foundation of all psycho-therapeutic success. No matter what form of mental disorder we are dealing with, and no matter what method of treatment we employ, the efficacy of all psycho-therapeutic endeavour depends on the occurrence of transference and the use made of the transference-relation after it has arisen. In treatment by suggestion the force inherent in the transference is directed against the symptoms and takes effect through the belief and compliance which are so readily given when the affections are engaged. A mere negation of the symptoms is here often sufficient to make them disappear. A hypnotist says to a paralyzed hysteric " now you can walk ", and the patient forthwith walks. Needless to say, this is not curing the hysteria, although it is bringing relief from the symptom. The paralysis will most probably be replaced by some other physical symptom or by some form of morbid anxiety. Yet it is not to be denied that there is something in the effects of suggestion thus used which still eludes understanding and which no theory of suggestion wholly explains. It is a difficulty related to the border-land between the mental and the physical, as when, in conversion hysteria, a painful affect seems to become converted into a bodily symptom. A similar problem is presented by the influence of suggestion on organic functions which are not under the control of the will, and in whose activity we might have supposed that belief or obedience could play no part. Yet, whatever may be the ultimate explanation of such organic compliance, we know that suggestion of its occurrence is ineffective in the absence of transference. In all other forms of pre-analytical treatment transference reveals itself in that personal influence of the physician which secures the acceptance of his explanations of the nature of the symptoms and the perseverance necessary to combat them, so long as the patient is assured of the physician's interest and support. But should he show any lack of interest or of willingness to help, or should any circumstances arise which tend to arouse the negative side of the transference so that the patient gets angry or annoyed with the physician, there comes an inevitable relapse and a recurrence or exacerbation of the symptoms. Treatment of neurosis by suggestion, by persuasion, or by re-education may, for this reason, become an intolerable burden to the physician and tends to keep the patient in a state of dependence on him which makes real recovery impossible so long as it lasts.

In treatment by all these methods a breaking of the transference is apt to be followed by a relapse into neurosis. In treatment by psycho-analysis the transference is made use of in an entirely different way, and getting free from the transference is the final step in getting free from neurosis. It is true that in treatment

by analysis the suggestibility inherent in the transference-situation is made use of, just as it is made use
of in these other methods ; but the personal influence
of the analyst is directed towards a totally different
end.   It is not directed against the symptoms, but is
wholly occupied in helping the patient to overcome the
resistances to self-knowledge.

The method of treatment specifically known as
psycho-analysis may be said to have been introduced
when Freud gave up using hypnosis for the purpose
of recovering the lost memories of neurotic patients,
and trusted entirely to free association in the waking
state.   From the beginning the therapeutic task was
recognized as an effort to bring back to consciousness
the unconscious impulses whose repression had led to
neurosis.   Attention was at first concentrated on a
search for the situations in the past life of the patient
which had determined the outbreak, and interpretation
of the material supplied by his free associations was
directed towards this end.   Resistance to the emergence
of what had been repressed was lessened by com-
municating the interpretations to the patient and by
insistence on the fundamental rule of psycho-analysis
that there must be no criticism or selection of the
incoming thoughts and that everything must be told.

In the present-day technique the analyst does not
concentrate on any particular element or problem
connected with the origin of the neurosis.   He devotes

his whole attention to what is occupying the patient's mind at the moment and to discovering the resistances which arise in connexion with it. Interpretation of the material supplied by the patient's conscious thoughts is directed towards discovering the unconscious resistances. When these are pointed out to the patient and surmounted, the forgotten memories may be recovered without difficulty.

The sole aim of analytic treatment is to bring back to consciousness the repressed impulses which are finding surrogate satisfaction in the symptoms, to restore the conflict between Ego and Libido to the conscious level, and to enable the patient to find some more satisfactory solution than that afforded by repression. The efforts of the analyst towards this end are helped by the transference; yet, strange to say, the transference is also the chief obstacle in the way of success. The transference in the searchlight of analysis is not the simple affective state that appears in other methods of treatment as confidence in, and devotion to, the physician. When subjected to analysis it is found to have its roots in erotic impulses which meet with great resistance when they try to enter consciousness. Moreover, the capacity for transference is not confined to positive love-relations; it shows itself also as a capacity for transferring to the analyst hostile feelings which had their origin in earlier experiences with other persons. Both of these aspects

of transference play a part in analysis, and both are
sources of resistance.   The negative transference, the
hostile feelings, are most frequently met with when the
patient is a man ; for he puts the analyst in his father's
place, and reproduces the feelings of antagonism to the
father which arose in his early life.   With women the
transference resistance more frequently takes the form
of tender and erotic feelings, and these also are derived
from the childhood attitude towards the father.   But
both hostile and erotic feelings enter into all analyses,
and are made use of by the resistance ; and in entering
into the resistance they supply important material
for analysis, without which, indeed, any deep
exploration of the unconscious is impossible.

Up to a certain point analysis by means of free
association leads to the recollection of much in the
patient's life that has a bearing on the onset and growth
of the neurosis ; but there comes a time when the
associations lead to the recall of affective attitudes
towards former love-objects, which are under strong
repression. The transference situation provides a means
of escape from these painful recollections, for now
the affect is displaced and instead of being revived
as a memory it is reproduced as an actual current
experience in relation to the analyst.   A man, for
example, cannot recall his hostile attitude towards
his father, but he adopts without any provocation a
hostile attitude towards the physican. A woman cannot

recall her childhood jealousy of her mother, but she confesses to an intense jealousy of the analyst's wife, whom she has never seen. The extent to which such repetition is substituted for recollection is a measure of the resistance to the recall of the repressed impulse, and the work of the analyst consists in translating the present experience into terms of the past, and removing the resistances which hinder recollection.

The regular occurrence of transference in every analysis of hysterical and obsessional patients is one of the strongest links in the chain of evidence which supports the Libido-theory of the neuroses. Its absence in our attempts to analyse persons suffering from melancholia, dementia praecox, or paranoia, is confirmatory of the hypothesis of narcissistic Libido and, in part, explanatory of the lack of therapeutic success which attends our efforts.

That transference must inevitably arise in the treatment of the transference-neuroses is a truth that was forced upon psycho-analysts and reluctantly accepted by them. At first it was thought it might be merely an accidental occurrence, and the analyst looked upon it as an unfortunate hindrance to the therapeutic work and a source of some annoyance to himself. But when, with fuller experience, it was found to occur in every case, no matter what sort of person the analyst was or what sort of person was being analysed, it became clear that it was no accident, but an essential

M

part of the neurosis. It is, indeed, what we may call
a new edition of the neurosis, and, when it is fully
developed, the therapeutic work is no longer concerned
with the original symptoms, but with the new
symptoms which consist in the various manifestations
of the transference. All the Libido which formerly
found satisfaction in the symptoms is now concentrated upon the person of the analyst, and in freeing
the patient from the transference he frees him from
neurosis.

The primary difficulty in dissolving the transference
is due to the resistances which hide from the patient
the true nature of the impulses on which it is based.
The overcoming of the resistances is effected by a
re-education of the Ego and by some modification of
the demands of the Ego-ideal. The Ego must accept
or be reconciled to libidinal impulses which formerly
had been summarily dealt with by repression. It must
learn that some degree of satisfaction of the Libido is
necessary, and it must effect some solution of the conflict other than repression ; for, if the resistances have
been overcome in the course of analysis, a retreat
of the Libido into the unconscious is no longer
possible.

The whole process of recovery is sometimes rendered
more difficult than it otherwise would be by that
seemingly constitutional peculiarity which has been
referred to as "adhesiveness of the Libido", i.e. the

difficulty of getting it freed from any object to which it has become attached.

A few days after I had received the invitation to deliver this course of lectures on Medical Psychology I asked a distinguished psychologist, a member of the Council, how much Freudian doctrine I might venture to expound to an audience drawn from members of the British Institute of Philosophical Studies. " Not much, I am afraid," he said, " you might deal with the general principles, but I don't think you can say much about—the Libido-theory, for example." For a moment I felt in a dilemma, but it soon became clear to me that the responsibility was not mine. If you want lectures on Medical Psychology at the present time you must be prepared to listen to Freudian doctrine ; and if you listen to Freudian doctrine you must hear about the Libido. It is as absurd to treat of Medical Psychology and leave out Freud, or to expound Freudian teaching and leave out the Libido, as it would be to play Hamlet without the Prince of Denmark.

As we have seen, the theory of the Libido forms the central core of Freud's teaching ; it is the foundation on which he built up his theory of the neuroses, and it enters into his explanation of the efficacy of all psycho-therapeutic measures. Just as the Libido, in repression, is the chief factor in the production of neurosis, so, in transference, it is the chief factor in the process of cure. Moreover, there is nothing in the theory of the

Libido or in the history of any of its phases, from which grown-up people need turn away. Like everything in life, it has a lowly origin, and in its beginnings it reveals itself in ways that are repudiated at the first glimmer of the dawn of culture and morality. In its final manifestations it enters into everything that is most valued in human life, and is the mainspring of all our most worthy activities ; it is the source of all desire, it is the spur to all. ambition, it is the root of all love. Its ultimate implications carry us far away from its naturalistic origins and enable us to keep company with those idealistic philosophers who hold love to be the greatest thing in the world.

SURVEY OF THE DOCTRINES OF MEDICAL
PSYCHOLOGY

IN surveying the contributions of Medical Psychology
to our knowledge of human nature, one of the
first questions that may be asked is, How far are the
doctrines derived from study of the neuroses applicable
to normal people ?   In considering this question we
need make no attempt to define precisely what we
mean by normal and abnormal.   There is obviously
no hard and fast line to be drawn between normal and
abnormal people or between normal and abnormal
behaviour. We use the word " normal " in a loose way
as indicating conformity to a rough average of healthy
mindedness such as characterizes the majority of the
people we meet every day ; and by an abnormal person
we mean one who has some neurotic or psychotic
disability which handicaps him, more or less, in the
tasks or enjoyments of life.

It will be convenient to deal separately with
the concepts of medical psychology which we
have distinguished as pre-Freudian and Freudian
respectively, and in connexion with the latter we may
refer to the opinions of certain writers whom I have
proposed to call post-Freudians. Of these the most
important are Alfred Adler and C. G. Jung, both of

whom were at one time psycho-analysts, but have since elaborated systems of their own which are subversive of psycho-analytic teaching. Adler calls his system Individual Psychology, and Jung has endeavoured to appropriate the term Analytical Psychology in order to distinguish his doctrines from those of Psycho-analysis properly so-called.

Besides these two workers and their followers, there is an influential group of psychologists in this country and America who have accepted to a greater or less extent the doctrines of Freud but are opposed to some of his views. This group is rather a heterogeneous one, for some of its members are opposed to Freud's views on matters that are fundamental to psycho-analytic theory and practice, whereas others only fail to follow Freud in what may be regarded as unessential or subsidiary portions of his teaching.

Now, just because there is no hard and fast line to be drawn between the normal and the abnormal, we must believe that the doctrines of medical psychology are in some degree applicable to all people. The peculiarities of mental functioning which we find well marked in the neuroses and psychoses are only exaggerations of modes of mental functioning that are common to all human beings. If we take, for example, the massive dissociations studied by Janet and Morton Prince, the well-marked cases of double personality, we know that we can find among so-called normal people incipient divisions of the self, temporary changes of character, alternations of mood, which are merely minor manifestations of the same order as those met with in definitely pathological conditions. Spontaneous or voluntary recovery from states of abstraction, ability to come back at need to full conscious awareness, seems to be all that distinguishes certain temporary dissociations from the more persistent dissociations of hysteria.

To this limited extent the theory of dissociation of pre-Freudian psychology finds some application in the life of normal people, but it cannot be said that such an application carries us very far. Nor does Janet's hypothesis of varying degrees of psychical tension enable us to understand the incidence of these minor dissociations ; it goes little beyond the everyday observation that these things are most likely to happen when one is, in popular language, " run down " or " below par ".

With the introduction of analytical methods in the investigation of abnormal states and the formulation of hypotheses to account for the facts thereby discovered, a noteworthy enlargement of the sphere of application of the doctrines of medical psychology took place. Almost every principle that has been invoked in explanation of abnormal mental process is found to be of equal value in the interpretation of normal behaviour. The part played by repression in

the life of the mind is now very widely acknowledged ;
the realm of the unconscious, whatever may be thought
of its nature or content, must be common to all ;
analytical theories of dream are as applicable to the
dreams of normal people as to those of neurotics ;
and the interpretation of the dreams of normal people
shows that their minds are fashioned on the same
pattern as those of their less fortunate fellows.

The light thrown by analytical doctrines upon the
working of the normal mind is one of the strongest
arguments in favour of the general truth of these
doctrines. Did they not contain much truth it is hardly
possible that hypotheses, put forward in explanation
of mental process and behaviour that are admittedly
abnormal, should be so illuminating when applied to
the workings of the normal mind and to the conduct
of normal people.

But what is revealed in the light thrown by psycho-
analysis on what goes on in the mind is not very pleasing
to man's self-esteem, and there have been many
desperate denials of the propriety of applying to normal
people the facts discovered in the analysis of those who
are abnormal. The terrible things that analysts find
in the unconscious of neurotics may be true of them,
it is said, but surely the minds of ordinary decent-
minded people are free from such evil desires and such
unnatural impulses !   Such denials may appear to
be rationally justified, but we know that in fact they

are always affectively determined. If you are told that in your unconscious you are a murderer or a thief, your whole being is immediately up in arms to defend yourself from so foul an imputation. That is the kind of reaction evoked in those who condemn psycho-analysis before they have begun to understand its teaching.

We do not expect to meet with a just appreciation of the truth or value of the doctrines of psycho-analysis from anyone who meets them for the first time. Rejection is inevitable, and the more " normal " one is, perhaps the more thorough and self-satisfied is the refusal to believe. But with patient study and a fuller knowledge many of the resistances to under-standing may be overcome, and an attitude of willing-ness to accept the truth, however unpalatable it may be, can be attained. Yet perhaps full conviction comes only to those who are brought to realize the truth in their personal experience, or who have the opportunity of discovering it by the actual analysis of other people. And even then the conviction may be more or less partial. Some of the conclusions of psycho-analysts are more easily accepted than others, and those that are almost self-evident to one person may seem most improbable to another. On the whole, it may be said that these differences are due to differences in the resistance, and depend very largely on the personal experiences of individuals and the environmental influences to which their lives have been subject.

But to say that all doubt or unbelief in relation to psycho-analytic teaching is due to resistance is to assume that everything taught by psycho-analysis is true. This would be a monstrous assumption, and Freud himself would be the last to make such a claim. For all through his work he has been his own most severe critic; time after time he has pointed out his own mistakes and abandoned positions he has held when he found they were no longer tenable in the light of fuller knowledge which his more extended experience brought him. But from the beginning there have been certain fundamental principles of his teaching which have remained unaltered and which wider experience has only more fully confirmed. These are the foundations of psycho-analytic theory, and it is the acceptance or the denial of these foundations that marks off the believer from the unbeliever in psycho-analysis.

Not long ago I was discussing psycho-analysis with an eminent psychiatrist who is still halting between two opinions in regard to it. " At least," I said, " you must admit it is a wonderful structure." " Yes," he replied, " I admit it is a wonderful structure, but it is not the structure I am troubling about, it is the foundations." And this is indeed a legitimate theme for scepticism and criticism ; although the fact that so great and complex a structure has been built up and has withstood for so long the many attacks that have been made upon it would lead us to suspect that the foundations cannot be so insecure as some criticisms of them might lead us to suppose.

It is not easy to decide what should be regarded as the bed-rock on which psycho-analysis rests. I am inclined to say that it is on the notion of mental conflict and repression. And it is instructive to observe that this fundamental feature of psycho-analytic theory is just the feature which is most widely accepted. The most orthodox of psychologists are constrained to accept this principle when they examine the data of medical psychology.

But repression as an outcome of conflict has little meaning unless we accept also the conception of the unconscious. We know that many psychologists reject altogether the notion of a mental unconscious ; and for those who do so the main conflicts with which psycho-analysis has to deal — the unconscious conflicts—can hardly be said to exist. It may well be then that belief in an unconscious region of the mind is also fundamental ; that the Unconscious is one of the foundation-stones of psycho-analysis. If an unconscious region of the mind is accepted as a corollory to the concepts of conflict and repression, we have in very general terms the frame-work of the plan on which psycho-analytic theory has been built up. We may imagine a part of the mind corresponding to the Freudian Ego and Ego-ideal, constantly at war with those instinctual tendencies, whatever they may be, which are unacceptable to the Ego, and which, as the issue of the conflict, are repressed in the unconscious.

But it may also be said that the kind of impulses that are repressed, or are most subject to repression, is also fundamental in psycho-analytic theory. And this, indeed, seems to be true. If we reject the Libido-theory and the doctrine of infantile sexuality, the whole structure which we know specifically as psycho-analysis tumbles to pieces, although we may still be left with a tenable view of the part played by conflict and repression in mental life, and with a possible theory of the neuroses.

Bound up with the conception of the Libido and not to be separated from it in psycho-analytic theory and practice is the doctrine of transference, and the hypothesis of displacement of affect which makes transference possible. These conceptions—conflict and repression, the unconscious, infantile sexuality, and transference—seem to me to be the fundamental conceptions of psycho-analysis, and anyone who accepts them may be said to accept psycho-analytic teaching.

Divergence of opinion is perhaps most likely to arise concerning the nature of the impulses that are subject to repression and the content of the unconscious. This is the point at which an influential body of English psychologists part company with Professor Freud and his followers. They accept the concepts of conflict, repression and the unconscious, and to some extent the doctrine of transference ; but they do not admit that only sexual impulses are repressed or that repressed sexual impulses alone are concerned in the development of neurosis. The late Dr. Rivers, who may well be regarded as the founder of this school, refused to follow Freud in this matter. His experience of the neuroses of war enabled him to investigate a large number of cases of hysteria and anxiety-states resulting from war-shock of one kind or another ; and although he was in many respects a most competent investigator and a firm believer in the psycho-analytical conceptions of conflict, repression, and the unconscious, he found no evidence that the war-neuroses, except in a small proportion of cases, were related in any way to the sexual instinct. He thought, however, " that these disorders became explicable as the result of disturbances of another instinct, one even more fundamental than that of sex— the instinct of self-preservation ; especially those forms of it which are adapted to protect the animal from danger,"[1] such as the instincts of flight and aggression. He ascribed war-neurosis to a conflict between the instincts of self-preservation and the call of duty, but he admitted the preponderance of sexual factors in the causation of the neuroses of civil life.

[1] Rivers, *Instinct and the Unconscious*, p. 5.

The problem presented by the war-neuroses has been
a stumbling block to many who were at first inclined
to accept the Libido-theory of the neuroses ; and their
difficulties seem to me to have been increased by the
too restricted conception of the Libido which is almost
forced upon our minds by the use of the word " sexual "
to describe every kind of tendency that can be called
libidinal.   The only way in which the war-neuroses
can be brought into line with psycho-analytic theory
is by invoking that disposition of the Libido which is
called narcissistic. But narcissistic Libido is desexualized
Libido ; conversion of object-Libido into Ego-Libido
involves   a   renunciation   of   sexual   aims—a desexualization.   Yet Ego-Libido is still Libido, and it is
the force underlying narcissism or self-love.   If we
recognize the libidinal side of self-preservation we need
no longer refuse to admit that the Libido-theory of
neurosis is applicable to the neuroses of war.

When Jung broke away from psycho-analysis his
belief in such a transformation of libido as that implied
in the process of desexualization was one of the indict-
ments in the charge of heresy brought against him by
orthodox Freudians.   At that time Freud had not, I
think,   laid   stress   upon   the   occurrence   of   desexualization, nor had he said much about instincts
inhibited in their aim, except in so far as such processes
are implicit in his doctrine of sublimation.   Jung's
heresy in this connexion, however, went farther than

merely teaching that Libido could become desexualized; he also taught that Libido is originally not sexual at all. He regarded the various instincts as issuing from an undifferentiated primal life-force, and to this primal life-force he unfortunately applied the term Libido. His doing so introduced a quite unnecessary confusion into a subject that was already sufficiently complicated. In childhood, he said, the Libido (in his sense) is almost wholly occupied in the instinct of nutrition, and sexuality is only its last and most important sphere of application. By applying the term Libido to the energy of the nutritional instinct he obliterates the important distinction between the nutritional element and the libidinal element (in the Freudian sense) in, for example, the act of sucking.

Another part of Jung's heresy was his division of the unconscious into a personal unconscious derived from individual experience and a collective unconscious which is a heritage from racial experience. The collective unconscious contains, in a condensed form, traces of the experience of the race; and this applies to modes of mental functioning as well as to mental content. Dream and phantasy in present-day man are but a regression to archaic modes of thought; the themes of myth and dream are the primordial images, the inherited potentialities of human imagination. Something approaching Jung's conception of the collective unconscious is implied, however, in Freud's acceptance of racial inheritance as the most reasonable explanation of what he calls typical dreams, typical symbols, and primal phantasies.

The heretical nature of Jung's departure from psycho-analytic doctrine becomes more apparent when we consider the slight emphasis he lays upon repression, and the nature and source of the conflict to which he attributes the occurrence of neurosis. The personal unconscious is not the result of repression following conflict but is merely a consequence of the tendency of every individual to develop one-sidedly in his mental growth. In adaptation to life one part of his potentialities is neglected in favour of the other and the neglected part tends to become unconscious. This doctrine, so subversive of psycho-analytic teaching, is part of Jung's theory of psychological types. When he first put forward his views on this topic he distinguished two types into which all human beings can be classed—the extrovert and the introvert. In the extrovert the fundamental function is feeling, in the introvert it is thought. In the extrovert the potentialities of thought tend to be unconscious, and in the introvert the potentialities of feeling tend to be unconscious,—just in so far as these potentialities are undeveloped in the conscious life.

According to Jung, some adaptations to life require more thought than feeling, while others require more feeling than thought ; and a conflict that may lead to neurosis arises when the introvert is faced by situations that demand feeling more than thought, or when the extrovert is called upon for more thought than feeling. It is a conflict between the function by which adaptation is ordinarily made, and the opposite function which through neglect has been allowed to become unconscious. Thus Jung has been led to give up looking for the cause of neurosis in the past life of the patient, and hopes to find it in the present. He asks, What is the necessary task in the patient's life which he will not fulfil and from which he recoils ? and his therapy is directed towards enabling the patient to recover the submerged function of feeling or of thought by which the necessary adaptation may be made. Moreover, Jung believes that the purposive nature of human striving is not confined to the conscious level, but is also found in the unconscious working of the submerged function. He thinks the unconscious attitude towards the tasks of life is revealed in dream, and in his interpretation of dreams he seeks for this revelation. The psyche as a whole reacts to the task in front of it, and what is missing in the conscious reaction is to be found in the unconscious. Only by combining the unconscious attitude with the conscious attitude is the most suitable solution of any of life's problems to be found.

Holding such views on the nature of the unconscious, Jung is unable to accept the Freudian interpretation

N

of sexual symbolism and phantasy. He does not regard sexual phantasies literally. He acknowledges the universal existence of the Oedipus complex, but he sees in the incest-wish no libidinal attitude towards the parent but merely a regressive revival of archaic modes of thought. An incest-phantasy is for him merely the means of expression used by the unconscious to indicate a need or desire for spiritual rebirth.

In their treatment of dream symbolism we see some of the fundamental differences between Freud and Jung in their outlook on human nature. Freud sets out from the assumption that the driving force behind all mental activity is the desire for pleasure and the avoidance of pain ; the gratification of desire is the primary aim of humanity and adaptation to the realities of life is a hard necessity imposed from without. Jung sees the primal Libido as a will-to-live ; adaptation to life, the fulfilment of a task, is the chief incentive : pleasure is obtained as a reward for duty done. As I have said elsewhere,[1] " Freud's outlook may be compared to that of Adam before the Fall—the pursuit of pleasure in a paradise of desire, marred only by the interdict placed upon the fruit of the forbidden tree. Jung's outlook is rather that of Adam after the expulsion from the garden, confronted with the task of adaptation if he would live."

From this brief summary of some of Jung's views,

[1] " Psychology of the Unconscious and Psycho-analysis," *Proceedings, S.P.R.* Vol. xxx, Part lxxv, p. 164.

we see that he rejects more than one of the foundation-stones of psycho-analysis. He hardly mentions repression, and he rejects the Freudian unconscious. He substitutes " neglect " for repression, and sees the conflict that leads to neurosis as a struggle, not between Ego and Libido, but between the adapted function and the unadapted function that lies to a great extent in the unconscious.

The view, accepted by Jung, that dreams are attempted solutions of the dreamer's current problems, was first put forward by Alfred Adler. For Adler, even more than for Freud or for Jung, all the activities of life are pervaded by purpose. But while for Freud the purpose is the attainment of pleasure and the avoidance of pain, while for Jung the purpose is adaptation to life, Adler would seem to see the whole purpose of life in the acquisition of power and superiority over one's fellows. At least he considers the desire for power and superiority to be the driving force in the life of the neurotic, in whom it becomes specially prominent as a reaction against feelings of inferiority.

Adler has shown that any inferiority or faulty development of bodily organs acts as a spur to persistent efforts to overcome the defect or its con-sequences, and to emulate those whom the child regards as superior or all-powerful. A feeling of inferiority, however brought about, leads to uncertainty and insecurity ; and, according to Adler, the whole purpose of life then becomes centred in a striving for

superiority and power.   When the attainment of this
goal is frustrated by the actualities of life, or when from
nature of the case it is an impossible or phantastic
goal, neurosis sets in ;   and the disabilities of the
neurosis are made use of as a means of continuing
the struggle for power.   They are put forward as
justification for the withdrawal from life which would
by itself point to inferiority and failure, and they
become the instruments of the dominance and
aggression which an invalid in a household can exercise
without fear of rebuff.

In opposition to the Freudian view of the all-
important part played by libidinal tendencies in the
production of neurosis, Adler lays all the stress on the
self-preservative or Ego-tendencies of aggression and
the " will-to-power ".   To attain a heightened Ego-
consciousness is the goal of the neurotic, and this
striving assumes the form of what Adler calls the
" masculine protest ".   The formula :   " I wish to be
a complete man," is, he says, the guiding fiction in
every neurosis.   He rejects entirely the sexual aetiology
of the neuroses and considers the sexual content of
neurotic phantasy to be merely an outcome of the
antithesis " masculine-feminine ", which originates
in the " masculine protest " ;   he says it is only a
" sexual jargon " which " must be regarded as symbolic
and requires interpretation ".

Although Adler was once a psycho-analyst, it is

even more true of him than of Jung that he has rejected the foundations of Freud's work. He does not recognize the unconscious, he makes no use of the concept of repression, and he rejects the theory of the Libido.

Thus we see that both Adler and Jung deny the fundamental principles on which Freudian doctrine is based ; and, whatever we may think of the systems they have raised on the foundations laid down by themselves, we cannot admit that their work has now any connexion with psycho-analysis. It is well to be clear about this, for it is a matter on which there seems to be widespread misunderstanding.

The position of those who, like Adler and Jung, reject the foundations on which psycho-analytic theory and practice have been built, is clearer in many ways than that of those who, like some of our English psychologists, accept some of the main principles of psycho-analysis and yet deny the validity of the conclusions arrived at by Freud and by those of his followers who are best fitted to form an opinion ; best fitted to form an opinion because they are actually doing the work through which alone, perhaps, real conviction can come.

In trying to appraise the truth and the value of psycho-analytic teaching we should, as in other departments of science, keep clearly before our minds the distinction between facts of observation and the inferences that may be drawn from them. But to do so is here more difficult than in the physical sciences. In psychology there are no facts of observation except those states of mind directly observed by introspection. We can, it is true, directly observe behaviour in other people, but our knowledge of the mental accompaniments of such behaviour is inferential. Less direct is the knowledge acquired from the introspective account given by another person of what is taking place in his mind. If we have reason to believe he is honest, and if what he tells us corresponds to something we have ourselves experienced, we accept his statements. In the forming of psychological hypotheses, knowledge thus acquired has to be reckoned as "facts of observation". In building up a theory of the workings of the mind we must rely mainly on these three ways of collecting facts : (1) introspection, (2) observation of behaviour, and (3) the introspective accounts given by those whose behaviour we observe.

These are the ways on which we rely in the study of the normal mind in its conscious and preconscious aspects ; and it is not otherwise when we study the abnormal mind or try to penetrate into the unconscious. But in trying to find in the unconscious of another person something that would correspond to a fact of observation, we are met by a difficulty which is peculiar to this field of investigation. Seeing that we have no direct knowledge of any mental states,

apart from introspection, we cannot realize or understand what another person tells us about his mental
states unless we have knowledge of similar states in
our own minds ; just as a person who is colour-blind
for " red " cannot understand what is meant by " red ".
So when we try to find out what is going on in the
unconscious of another person, we are entirely baffled
unless we have direct or immediate knowledge of similar
events in our own unconscious. Every one of our own
repressions forms a blind spot in our mental apparatus ;
and thus it comes about that what psycho-analysts
tell us they have discovered in the unconscious is so
widely denied or disbelieved.

Although this difficulty, due to our own repressions,
provides a barrier which effectually prevents any wide
acceptance of the doctrines of psycho-analysis, nevertheless, as we have seen, some of the fundamental
conceptions of the method are now very generally
admitted ; and it is probably only a matter of time
for some of the others to pass the individual and social
censorship which prompts to unbelief.

It is sometimes objected that the facts of observation
in psycho-analysis—the material supplied by the
person undergoing analysis—are distorted by the
method of investigation employed, and that the nature
of this material is influenced by the preconceptions of
the analyst. Considerations of this kind have induced
Dr. Bernard Hart, in his Goulstonian Lectures, to

cast doubt on the scientific validity of the method of psycho-analysis. His contention is that the facts of observation are not simple facts of observation such as are dealt with in the physical sciences, but are liable to distortion by the method used in discovering them. That this objection is not valid may be proved by anyone who undertakes an analysis and secures adherence to the one fundamental rule of the method, namely, that the patient tells *everything* that comes to the surface of consciousness. If association is allowed free play, and no criticism or selection of the incoming thoughts is exercised, the "facts of observation" presented will correspond to those described by the psycho-analysts.

It is hardly reasonable, however, for Dr. Hart to contrast the method of psycho-analysis with the methods of physical science ; and probably every form of psychological investigation would come equally badly out of such a comparison. We should be content if the methods of psycho-analysis conform to the principles of science in so far as these are applicable to psychology, and if the methods of science are adhered to in the interpretation of the facts observed.

To many it would seem that the most justifiable doubts concerning psycho-analysis arise in respect of the method of interpretation and the hypotheses put forward to account for the facts observed, rather than in respect of the possibility of distortion of the facts themselves. Of the many hypotheses that have been put forward to explain and correlate the facts of psycho-analysis, those that have longest stood the test of time, and explain the greatest number of phenomena, should obtain the greatest credence. As we get farther and farther away from these well-founded hypotheses we rightly get more and more cautious in giving our assent ; and there are at the present time, in the writings of psycho-analysts, many speculations that cannot be regarded as necessary parts of the theory of psycho-analysis.

Freud himself has plainly recognized the danger of such speculations. There are certain ideas which cannot be worked out, he says, " except by combining facts with pure imagination many times in succession, and thereby departing far from observation. We know that the final result becomes the more untrustworthy the oftener one does this in the course of building up a theory, but the precise degree of uncertainty is not ascertainable. One may thereby have made a brilliant discovery, or one may have gone ignominiously astray." [1] As an example we might take Freud's own speculations on life-instincts and death-instincts or his division of the mind into the Id, the Ego, and the Ego-ideal. All recent psycho-analytical writings make use of these speculations and of the new terminology introduced by Freud. Yet I venture to

[1] *Beyond the Pleasure Principle*, p. 77.

think that these conceptions do not at present form an essential part of psycho-analytic theory, however useful they may be for purposes of exposition. To quote Freud's own words in another connexion, " these ideas are not the basis of the science upon which everything rests ; that, on the contrary, is observation alone. They are not the foundation-stone, but the coping of the whole structure, and they can be replaced and discarded without damaging it." (*Collected Papers*, iv, p. 34.)

I have taken psycho-analysis as the main theme of these lectures because it is the dominating influence in all the work on Medical Psychology that is being done in this country at the present time. It is the centre around which all other schools of mental pathology and mental therapeutics revolve.   Those who are hostile to many of its tenets cannot get away from it, although they cannot accept it. It thus remains a force which has important effects far beyond the range of influence exerted by the relatively small group of workers who unreservedly acknowledge themselves adherents.

Belief in its doctrines is not easily or lightly acquired, and rejection of them is often accompanied by so much scorn and by such evidence of self-satisfied superiority as should warn us of the affective basis of such judgments. On the other hand, it may be thought that some of Freud's adherents are too scornful of the objections to their views that have been put forward from many quarters.   Some justification for this attitude may be found when it is realized that by far the greater part of the published opposition and criticism is founded on ignorance—ignorance of the facts on which psycho-analysis is based and ignorance of the elements of psycho-analytic theory as it really is. When people do not, or cannot, or will not understand what to us may seem self-evident truth, we are apt to turn away from them in the spirit of Abt Vogler, when he said : " The rest may reason and welcome : 'tis we musicians know." And this is an attitude which, in the field of Medical Psychology, is not confined to any one school. There is a sort of intellectual arrogance which sometimes comes with deep conviction, and it may lead the members of opposed schools to unseemly insistence on the rightness of their own particular doctrines. Then, like rival tradesmen, puffing their own merchandise, each school puts over its portals a sign-board with this notice :

> " Here truth is sold, the only genuine ware ;
> See that it has our trade mark ! you will buy
> Poison instead of food across the way."

Let us avoid all such vain assertions, for truth is many sided. Observers stationed at different points along the sea-shore, when the moon is up, all see a ray of moonlight on the water ; but no one observer can see, from where he stands, the light that seems so brilliant to his neighbour. So it may be that those who wrongly deny that any light is to be found where we are looking may yet themselves see some aspect of the truth which is hidden from our vision.

INDEX